Research for Evidence-Based Practice in Healthcare

This edition first published 2011
© 2011 and 2006 by Robert Newell and Philip Burnard

Blackwell Publishing was acquired by John Wiley & Sons in February 2007.
Blackwell's publishing program has been merged with Wiley's global
Scientific, Technical, and Medical business to form Wiley-Blackwell.

Registered office:
John Wiley & Sons Ltd, The Atrium, Southern Gate, Chichester, West Sussex,
PO19 8SQ, UK

Editorial offices:
9600 Garsington Road, Oxford, OX4 2DQ, UK
2121 State Avenue, Ames, Iowa 50014-8300, USA

For details of our global editorial offices, for customer services and for
information about how to apply for permission to reuse the copyright material
in this book please see our website at www.wiley.com/wiley-blackwell.

The right of the author to be identified as the author of this work has been
asserted in accordance with the UK Copyright, Designs and Patents Act 1988.

Library of Congress Cataloging-in-Publication Data

Newell, Robert, 1954–
    Research for evidence-based practice in healthcare/Robert Newell, Philip
Burnard. – 2nd ed.
        p. ; cm. – (Vital notes)
    Rev. ed. of: Vital notes for nurses : research for evidence-based
practice/Robert Newell, Philip Burnard. 2006.
    Includes bibliographical references and index.
    ISBN 978-1-4443-3112-7 (pbk. : alk. paper)
    1. Nursing–Research–Methodology.   2. Evidence-based nursing.
I. Burnard, Philip.   II. Newell, Robert, 1954- Vital notes for nurses.   III. Title.
IV. Series: Vital notes.
    [DNLM: 1. Nursing Research–methods.   2. Evidence-Based Nursing–
methods. WY 20.5 N546r 2011]
    RT81.5.N46   2011
    610.73072–dc22

                                                                    2010011213

A catalogue record for this book is available from the British Library.

Set in 10/12pt Palatino by Aptara® Inc., New Delhi, India
Printed and bound in Malaysia by Vivar Printing Sdn Bhd
1   2011

Contents

Additional resource material can be found on the book's website at:
www.wiley.com/go/newell

List of Common Research Terms

Case study	A descriptive approach to research involving multiple sources of information about a person, organisation or other entity
Content analysis	The organisation and categorisation of text material
Descriptive statistics	Quantitative data analysis approach used to simplify presentation of data from a given sample
Ethnography	Qualitative research method involving study of a culture
Evidence-based practice	An approach to clinical problem solving involving a systematised synthesis of available information
Experiment	Quantitative research method involving randomisation, manipulation of an independent variable, use of a control group
Findings	The outcomes of the analysis of qualitative research (occasionally used broadly to mean any kind of results in a research study)
Four principles approach to ethics	Approach emphasising; respect for autonomy; beneficence; non-maleficence; justice

Hypothesis	Explicit statement of the predicted relationship between independent and dependent variables
Inferential statistics	Quantitative data analysis approach used to draw inferences from sample data to its population
Phenomenology	Qualitative research method involving examination of people's perceptions of their experiences
Qualitative research	Broad approach to research emphasising analysis of text material
Quantitative research	Broad approach to research emphasising analysis of numerical material
Quasi-experiment	Quantitative research method similar to an experiment but with control and/or random assignment missing
Randomised controlled trial	A type of experiment used to investigate effectiveness of therapeutic interventions
Reliability	The extent to which a quantitative study examines the entity it says it does in a consistent and repeatable way
Respondents	Those who are studied or take part in a qualitative study
Results	The outcomes of the analysis of quantitative research
Sampling	Process by which subjects are chosen to participate in a research project
Single case experiment	Application of experimental and quasi-experimental methods to a single individual
Subjects	People whose responses are researched by researchers, in quantitative studies. Participants in research other than the researchers themselves
Systematic review	Systematised, rigorous approach to literature search and review
Validity	The extent to which a study examines the entity it says it does

SECTION 1
Contextual Materials

Introduction to Healthcare Research for Evidence-Based Practice

Introduction

This book is about research in healthcare, seen principally from the viewpoint of students undertaking pre-registration and post-registration educational programmes. We are both active healthcare researchers and are passionate believers in research by healthcare professionals (HCPs)[1] for the benefit of the patients and clients we serve. Our own background is principally in mental health nursing, although, as teachers and researchers, we have widened the scope of our work beyond a purely mental health focus. Likewise, as researchers we have typically worked in multidisciplinary research, with the broad range of other HCPs, with medical practitioner researchers and with researchers from a range of non-clinical disciplines. In preparing this book, we have sought to make it relevant to colleagues from across the disciplines, and we hope this comes over in the material that follows. We both started to get interested in research from early on in our clinical careers, and did a good deal of research while still mainly working as clinicians. The real reason we started in research was because we were interested in whether the things we did with patients and clients made a difference to their experiences of illness, recovery and health. If you have picked up this book, we guess you have a similar interest, and we hope we can work with you in developing that interest and finding ways you can translate your ideas into practical projects, whether these be through

Research for Evidence-Based Practice in Healthcare, Second edition, by Robert Newell and Philip Burnard
© 2011 Robert Newell and Philip Burnard

your own research or your examination of the research literature to inform your practice.

In the following pages, we will try and take you through the various elements of undertaking a piece of research. Even if you do not have to do research yourself as part of your educational course, this book is still for you for three reasons. First, much of the material we present is *essential*, not just for doing your own research, but for understanding the research of others. Because almost all healthcare courses these days require you to critically appraise the research that is already out there, you need an understanding of how to do that. Books and articles which just deal with critical appraisal are fine, as far as they go, but you will certainly have a much better understanding of how to evaluate published research if you have a clear idea of the various elements that go into a research project, the methods used by researchers and the reasoning behind methodological choices they have made. This book will give you that information.

Second, you will almost certainly encounter, during your course or later, the need to undertake some project work, for example developing a new guideline or a new way of organising care. All the information given here will help you to organise and evaluate that project.

Finally, a great deal of clinical practice is investigated by medical practitioners and non-clinical researchers, partly because comparatively few HCPs other than medical practitioners go on to become full-time researchers. We want to increase the number that do, so that HCPs are increasingly responsible for evaluating their own practice and get the credit for doing so. Ultimately, we would like you to be in a position to decide you want to be one of those people, so part of the job of this book is to give you a taste of what is involved, including some of its complexities, so that you will want to go on and find out more. We believe that research is essentially a practical skill and is best learnt through an apprenticeship system, and so the best piece of advice we can give you is to get hold of someone who has experience of actually doing research, translating research into practice, doing a systematic review and so on, and learn from them.

Then, use this book as your workshop guide. If you cannot find such an experienced researcher, then we hope this book will be able to tell you some of the things they would have. The book is not heavily referenced (usually only a few per chapter), but each of the references is important, and is easily available, either from your library or from the internet. We have made considerable use of web sources so as to make it easy for you to find the best supporting information. We know web sources do not necessarily remain current forever, but we believe the best ones do. When we came to write the second edition of this book, we found only a few sites that were no longer available.

The scope of healthcare research

Until quite recently, healthcare research had a reputation for being an introspective pursuit which was more concerned with investigating its own workforce than undertaking clinical research. Some commentators have suggested that becoming a teacher of healthcare professionals frequently involved ceasing to have any clinical responsibility for patient care or, indeed, much contact with clinical settings at all. In consequence, those teachers wishing to do research had little access to patients or were often out of touch with issues which were important to patients. They did, however, have contact with students, and so ended up developing research interests related to education and the views and experiences of student nurses. Sometimes, it was difficult to see how this research would benefit patients. Although this criticism was chiefly aimed at nurse researchers, our experience with the broad range of healthcare professionals suggests it holds true equally in other disciplines, a belief reinforced by the fact that initiatives to increase research by non-medical health disciplines have typically been applied across the range of disciplines.

We do believe that healthcare research is changing for the better, though, and is nowadays much more concerned with patient care, rather than being overly inward looking towards its own professions. Whilst we recognise that it is important for research to be done into such things as the opinions and experiences of students and members of the healthcare professions, or the ways in which these professionals are educated, we also think that the eventual point of all healthcare research should be the greater good of patients. Therefore, we suggest, the vast bulk of research into such issues as the views of the professions themselves should have immediate consequences for patient care. If it does not, then why do we want healthcare researchers doing it, rather than, say, sociologists or educationalists? Surely, examination of, for example, occupational therapists' opinions of their educational preparation, can be done as well by researchers from other disciplines. Given that healthcare researchers are a rare breed, we hope that the growing focus on clinical research, where nurses can make a distinctive contribution, will continue.

That said, many people are largely unaware of the contributions to research that healthcare professionals have made already, or the effect which that research has had on care. Just two fairly random examples from our own areas of interest give an idea of the scope of research by healthcare professionals. Professor Mary Jo Dropkin, from the University of Long Island, has written definitive studies of the psychosocial impact of head and neck cancer. Her work is cited by researchers across the whole range of health disciplines and has changed the way we think about head and neck cancer. In the UK, Professor Trudie Chalder from

Kings College, London, is a world-recognised expert in fatigue, and developed the leading mode of treatment in this area. Once again, her work is referred to by all the healthcare professions. When you consider that fatigue is cited as a major symptom in almost all long-term physical conditions, it is easy to see the extent of this HCP's contribution to the potential well-being of patients via her research.

Whose business is research in healthcare?

As you can tell from the above, we think it is primarily the business of HCPs themselves to evaluate and develop our care through research. These days, almost all large-scale research is undertaken in teams, and almost all these teams are multidisciplinary. All HCPs need to be equipped to take a full part in these teams. In the past, we have been ill equipped to do so, and, given the packed nature of healthcare pre-registration education, research often takes a back seat. As we said above, very few clinicians go on to be full-time researchers, but all of us are research *users*, even when we are not aware of it. Being a *knowledgeable, aware* consumer of research findings is integral to competent practice.

Apart from using research in our own clinical practice, we have a further ethical obligation concerning use of research, and one which exceeds the responsibility of members of the general public. For example, HCPs need to be sufficiently knowledgeable about research to help patients who may become involved in research projects run by other members of the clinical team to make reasonable, informed choices about, for example, participation in such a study. Similarly, patients may ask our views about treatment which is currently practiced, and we are unable to offer such advice without an informed understanding of the evidence base. This, in turn, comes from an understanding of the research approaches which have been used to generate this evidence.

Surprisingly, even in everyday life, away from clinical practice, our role as an HCP gives us a greater ethical obligation to understand the evidence behind healthcare interventions, because our role may give us a certain amount of authority when we communicate (even very informally) with others about healthcare matters and healthcare research. Accordingly, we have a special responsibility to ensure that we know what we are talking about. This implies, once again, a knowledge of research methods.

Which brings us to our final point in this section. Very little healthcare has been subject to robust clinical research. This leaves us, we believe, with two important responsibilities. First, we should be basing our care as far as possible on the best available evidence. This implies an ability to search for, appraise and implement that evidence. Appraisal requires a basic understanding of the merits of the studies we read, and a knowledge of research methods is essential to that understanding. Second, the knowledge base needs building, so involvement, at whatever level, in research to build it is as part of our ethical responsibility as HCPs in just the same way as use of current best evidence.

Perhaps the key questions at the heart of evidence-based practice in the health professions are as follows:

What works?
What works best?
How does it work?

Research provides a starting point in answering these questions.

Using this book to get involved in healthcare research

We want this book to be a practical guide. Part of being practical is being as easy to access as possible. This leaves us with a problem. We have tried to make each chapter as stand-alone as possible, but at the same time we wanted to avoid repetition, so we do not go over every piece of background information necessary in each chapter. This means there will inevitably be some shifting around for you between chapters, and we hope you will dip in and out to follow up things we have not been able to cover over and over again as they occur in different contexts. To help you do this, we are going to avoid giving you the traditional detailed chapter-by-chapter description of what is going to be covered in this book. Instead, here we are simply giving you each chapter title, followed by the key points section for that chapter. As a result, at any point, you will be able to flick back to this chapter (dog ear it now) and read through key points to give you an idea of where relevant issues are covered. Please do not feel you have to read the whole book. It is a tool. Use what you need and leave the rest. Maybe it will be of use later.

The chapters

Chapter 2: The research process – organising your research

The research process is a way of organising a research project.
The study aims and objectives guide the study.
The literature review provides the context for the study and determines the need for it.
All stages of the process should be clearly described with appropriate rationale.
Issues of ethics are fundamental to the research process.
Dissemination and implementation complete the research process and start the research cycle with new questions.

Chapter 3: Choosing methodological approaches

Researchers tend to associate inductive reasoning with qualitative research and theory building, and deductive reasoning with quantitative research and theory testing.

Quantitative approaches emphasise cause–effect relationships and prediction.

Qualitative approaches emphasise exploration.

Researchers should examine the goals of their research when choosing methodological approaches.

Consider qualitative approaches first for studies of individuals' experiences; research with excluded and hard to reach groups; pilot studies.

Consider quantitative approaches first for epidemiological studies of large groups; treatment comparison studies.

Chapter 4: Searching the literature

Literature searches are done primarily to ensure awareness of a field of research.

Systematic reviews examine the literature using systematised, transparent criteria.

A search strategy consists of the research question, its components, sources of information, search terms, retrieval and inclusion criteria, available resources.

Sensitivity (recall) refers to comprehensivity of a search strategy.

Specificity (precision) refers to relevance of a search strategy.

The scope of a search is determined by its search strategy.

Chapter 5: Ethics of healthcare research

Codifications of research ethics date from the Nuremberg code and the declaration of Helsinki.

Autonomy, beneficence, non-maleficence and justice are key principles in research ethics.

Autonomy refers to an individual's freedom to choose and act.

Beneficence and non-maleficence require that we maximise good and minimise harm.

Justice is the maximising of fairness to all.

Research ethics committees exist to interpret these concepts for the protection of research participants and researchers.

All research should receive ethical scrutiny.

All NHS-related research must receive approval from a Research Ethics Committee (REC).

NHS REC approval is centrally organised and standardised.

All NHS research must receive Research Governance approval from the NHS institution in which it takes place.

Research Governance approval is locally organised by each institution and there is limited standardisation.

Chapter 6: Basic concepts – sampling, reliability and validity

Sampling is an everyday activity, not peculiar to research.

A population is a total group from which a sample is drawn.

Some populations are themselves samples from larger populations

Representativeness is key to sampling, but is defined differently by quantitative and qualitative researchers.

Samples may be random or non-random.

Sampling technique is guided by the aim of the research.

Validity is the extent to which a study examines the entity it says it does.

Reliability is that it does so in a systematised, repeatable way.

Quantitative and qualitative researchers place different emphasis on different aspects of validity and reliability.

Chapter 7: Issues in qualitative data collection

Data collection choices are made in response to research aims.

Sampling in qualitative research aims at illumination rather than representativeness.

Interviews may be structured, semi-structured or unstructured.

Interviews are normally transcribed verbatim.

Sometimes, qualitative data can be gleaned from questionnaires.

Observational studies benefit from painstaking field notes.

Published work can be subjected to similar data analysis to other research methods.

Chapter 8: Case studies

Case studies are descriptive pieces of qualitative research.

Case studies may be stand-alone investigations or illustrations from larger studies.

Case studies examine a particular person, group, situation or set of circumstances in detail.

Case studies are not necessarily typical of general experiences.

Case studies rely on a high level of detailed description.

Sample selection for case studies can lead to challenges in terms of typicality or inevitable comparisons with other settings.

Chapter 9: Ethnography

Ethnography involves the in-depth study of a culture.

Ethnographic approaches use elements of ethnography.

Ethnographic approaches can be combined with other methods.

Ethnographic approaches usually involve extended amounts of field work.

Ethnography combines observation with other methods such as interviews.

Formal recording of interviews may often be impossible, so field notes are particularly important.

Disconfirming evidence is actively sought.

The range of phenomena to be observed is potentially overwhelming.

Ethnography reminds us of the importance of cultural context.

Chapter 10: Phenomenology

Phenomenology is concerned with individuals' perceptions of their experiences.

Phenomenology as a philosophy is concerned with seeing things without making value judgements.

Phenomenology frequently uses in-depth interviews and series of interviews.

Bracketing is the attempt to put aside one's own thoughts, feelings and beliefs.

The researcher avoids explanations of people's accounts so that the person's own voice can emerge.

Phenomenology aims to create vivid personal insights.

Chapter 11: A pragmatic approach to qualitative data analysis

Content analysis refers to the organising and ordering of textual material.

Transcription involves writing out recordings of an interview.

Some degree of quantification is possible.

Categories can be pre-defined or can emerge from the data.

The pragmatic approach involves six stages:
- taking memos after each interview
- reading transcripts and making notes of general themes
- repeated reading and generating open coding headings to describe all aspects of the data
- reducing the codes under higher order headings
- returning to the data with the higher order codes
- collating the organised data for reporting

Chapter 12: Limitations of qualitative research

Qualitative research does not claim to be scientific in the same way as quantitative research.

Samples in qualitative research are rarely representative.

The researcher's own influence on the emerging data may be checked by bracketing and by discussion with respondents.

There is too much variability to allow replication of qualitative studies.

Qualitative research does not aim to generalise.

Neither researcher nor respondent is necessarily aware of their own biases.

Analysis of interviews can be affected by hindsight bias.

Validation by respondents is itself potentially problematic.

Respondents can offer explanations about things they have no way of knowing about.

The illuminative value of quantitative research is slowly gaining ground in healthcare.

Chapter 13: Sampling, reliability and validity issues in data collection and analysis

Random sampling decreases the likelihood that members of a sample are different from its population.

Stratification and cluster sampling both ensure adequate representation of population subgroups in a sample.

Quota sampling and systematic sampling approximate to random sampling.

Convenience sampling is the simplest form of sampling but is least likely to conform to its population.

External validity refers to the applicability of a study to the real world.

Population validity refers to the similarity between a study sample and its population.

Ecological validity refers to the similarity between study conditions and procedures and the real world.

Internal validity determines the confidence we can have in cause–effect relationships in a study.

Reliability consists of two concepts: consistency and repeatability.

Consistency implies that, if a phenomenon is unchanged, it will be measured as the same by several observers or by several measuring methods.

Repeatability means that, if a phenomenon is unchanged, it will be measured as the same on several occasions.

Chapter 14: Cause and effect, hypothesis testing and estimation

Assertions about cause and effect are probabilistic, not definitive.

We make cause–effect predictions in daily life.

Cause–effect predictions in healthcare research are the same as those in daily life.

Quantitative researchers are concerned with independent variables, dependent variables and intervening variables.

Researchers manipulate independent variables, observe any changes to dependent variables and attempt to account for intervening variables.

Hypotheses are explicit statements of the predicted relationship between independent and dependent variables.

Directional hypotheses are made only when there is reason to think a relationship operates only in one direction.

Adequate statistical power is essential to the safe acceptance of the null hypothesis.

Hypothesis testing is an all-or-nothing statement of relatedness, but estimation emphasises the extent of a relationship.

Chapter 15: Experimental and quasi-experimental approaches

Experiments consist of three elements: manipulation of the independent variable, use of a control group, random allocation to experimental conditions.

These three elements allow experiments to claim a high degree of internal validity.

Quasi-experimental designs use a similar *general* approach to true experiments but control and/or random assignment may be missing.

Repeated measures approaches use the same participants for all experimental conditions.

Repeated measures approaches are vulnerable to order effects.

Order effects may be reduced by counterbalancing.

Independent groups designs use different participants for different experimental conditions.

Independent groups designs without randomisation are vulnerable to differences in participant characteristics (subject variability).

Matched pairs designs match participants on important variables to combat subject variability.

Factorial designs study interactions between several different independent variables.

Chapter 16: The single case experiment

Single case experiments apply experimental methods to treatment of single individuals.

Single case experiments allow you to do research in the course of clinical practice.

In AB designs and variants, different interventions are introduced and withdrawn sequentially.

In multiple baseline designs, responses to different interventions are compared cross-sectionally.

Systematised measurement is essential to single case experiments.

Data analysis is often confined to visual inspection of changes in scores.

Visual inspection can involve examining raw scores, means, levels, trends and latencies.

Statistical approaches have been developed because the interpretation of visual data can be subject to bias.

Single case experiments have good internal validity but poor external validity.

Chapter 17: Randomised controlled trials

A randomised controlled trial (RCT) is a type of experiment.

RCTs involve randomisation, a control group and manipulation of the independent variable.

RCTs attempt to control bias.

RCTs are the most effective way of examining cause and effect relationships, including the effect of treatment on patients.

Explanatory trials possess high internal validity and establish what principle, mechanism or theory accounts for a change in patient condition.

Pragmatic trials possess high external validity and establish how well a principle, a mechanism or a theory translates into the real clinical world.

RCTs are essential in providing patients with accurate information about healthcare interventions.

Chapter 18: Non-experimental approaches

Non-experimental approaches involve observation of naturally occurring relationships and differences between variables.

Non-experimental approaches are useful when experimental approaches are unethical or impractical.

Causal inference is weak in non-experimental approaches.

Descriptive designs only describe relationships between variables.

Causal–comparative designs (comparative/ex post facto designs) compare two or more naturally occurring groups.

Correlational designs explore relationships between variables in a single group.

Some correlational approaches allow prediction through the assignment of predictor variables.

Chapter 19: Surveys

Surveys are often wrongly assumed to be simple to carry out properly.

Sampling technique and sample size are important in determining the margin of error in a survey.

Survey designs are typically observational, but may also use experimental and quasi-experimental approaches.

Decisions about question construction and questionnaire administration are fundamental to a successful survey.

A recent systematic review has revealed that some 'research folklore' guidelines about survey methods and question construction are not supported by empirical research.

Chapter 20: The role of statistics

Statistics are important because they convey large amounts of data in an understandable way.

Statistics describe data and allow us to draw inferences based on probability from these data.

Data are divided into continuous (ratio, interval, ordinal) and categorical (nominal/categorical) data.

Statistical tests are divided into parametric and non-parametric tests.

Parametric tests usually assume data are at interval level, normally distributed and possess homogeneity of variance.

Different statistical tests are designed to deal with different types of data.

Different tests are designed to deal with different sources of variability from different research designs.

Chapter 21: Evidence-based practice and clinical effectiveness

Research aims to add to the evidence to inform clinical practice.

Evidence-based practice (EBP) and clinical effectiveness are related terms, but clinical effectiveness has the narrower focus.

EBP is a process involving asking answerable questions, finding evidence, appraising the evidence, applying evidence to practice, evaluating performance of EBP.

The hierarchy of evidence runs from most to least trustworthy on the basis of freedom from bias.

EBP is intended to enhance clinical decision-making, not replace it.

Chapter 22: Critical evaluation of research reports

The ability to weigh evidence is a required skill for competent practitioners.

A good literature review should critically examine the literature and set the current study in that context.

The method section should be detailed and demonstrate appropriate choices.

Different specific methodological issues are associated with qualitative and quantitative research.

The results section should be clear.

Quantitative results should distinguish between significant and non-significant results.

Qualitative results should avoid claims as to generalisability.

The discussion section should set the results in the context of the literature, implications for practice and further research.

Study weaknesses should be honestly and comprehensively reported.

Chapter 23: Writing a research report

The report is a product – help the reader.

All reports follow a similar general structure.

The executive summary is all most readers will read.

Do not spend too long on general methodological debate.

When reporting results:
- be clear
- be comprehensive
- distinguish clearly between results and comment

A good discussion amplifies the study results, shows the importance of the study results, relates the results to earlier research and theory, admits shortcomings of the study, shows implications for future research and for practice.

Follow assignment or journal guidelines exactly.

Write with short words, sentences and paragraphs.

Use linking sentences to join paragraphs.

Avoid punctuation you do not understand.

Write in written English, not spoken English.

Read work aloud to help with punctuation.

Chapter 24: Getting research into practice

The theory of diffusion of innovation divides change adopters into innovators, early adopters, early and late majority, and laggards.

Change diffusion is mediated by personal characteristics and accessibility of the innovation.

Journal articles are ineffective in changing practice.

A clear dissemination and implementation strategy should be devised on the basis of a diagnostic analysis.

The analysis should inform broad-based interventions to introduce the change.

The BARRIERS scale identifies four elements of barriers to change the adopter, the organisation, the innovation and the communication.

Notes on person and gender

We wrote this book together, with the idea of a series of conversations with you, the reader, in mind. For that reason, it is written largely in the first person plural, and we often address you directly. Occasionally, we vary this slightly and use the first person singular. This is usually to recount something which has happened to one of us and which has influenced our development as individuals and as researchers. Really, this is just to avoid cumbersome expressions like 'one of the authors (RN)' and so on. We hope this direct style is one you can engage with and will help you get into the spirit of a conversation with us about research.

We have made no definite choice about the use of the personal pronoun, and we refer to he or she pretty much indiscriminately throughout the book.

Good luck with this book and your research.

Endnote

1. Throughout this book, we will use the expression 'Healthcare Professionals' to refer to the broad range of clinical professions in healthcare (e.g. nurses, midwives, physiotherapists, occupational therapists, radiographers, podiatrists, clinical prosthetists and many, many others). We are excluding medical practitioners from this category for no other reason than that their educational and clinical tradition has developed very differently, and led to a different (and, perhaps greater) preparation for and engagement with the research that provides evidence for practice.

The Research Process – Organising Your Research

Introduction

This book is about all aspects of the research process as it relates to healthcare research. This chapter offers an overview of what is involved in that process and can be read in conjunction with other, more specific, chapters. Those chapters will, for example, discuss the differences between qualitative and quantitative approaches to research. Whatever

Research for Evidence-Based Practice in Healthcare, Second edition, by Robert Newell and Philip Burnard
© 2011 Robert Newell and Philip Burnard

approach is chosen, the same broad process is undertaken and it is this broad process that is under discussion here. Many writers have described the research process, often providing subtly different components. We do not subscribe to any one description of the process rather than another. Instead, we offer below a series of suggestions as to how a research project might be organised, based on the following view of the research cycle: research questions, literature review, selection of sample, selection of measures, data collection, data analysis, report writing and dissemination. Indeed, much of this book is constructed with this cycle in mind.

In a way, research is always a cyclical process. Once findings from a study have been established, they nearly always bring us back to new questions that need answering. It is not a good idea to view research as establishing 'the truth'. It is merely offering the best view we have on a given topic at a particular time in history.

The title

A research project needs a descriptive title. When other researchers are looking to see what research has been done before, it is the title of the project that will alert them, either to want to read the report of that project or to pass over it. The title, then, should be concise and, as clearly as possible, describe the nature and content of the research project. Thus, a title such as:

> *'A qualitative study of student midwives' views of reflective practice'*

is preferable to:

> *'The mirror of the mind: students and reflective practice'*

The first title states clearly both the nature and the content of the study, whilst the second one is less clear. It is probably best to avoid what might be called 'romantic' titles, or titles that use an analogy (such as 'The mirror of the mind...'), as these may be confusing or may miss the point. The title, wherever possible, should indicate both the research approach used *and* the topic of the study.

The title should, until the research is finished, be considered a 'work in progress'. It may be found that the title changes as the study is completed. Considerable time should be given to ensuring that the title is as accurate and as concise as possible. It is usually intimately related to the research questions.

The abstract

One of the final tasks in designing a research project is to write an abstract for the study. It is discussed here because it is usually one of the first pages in a research report or proposal for funding. An abstract is normally a one-page description of all aspects of the study. Thus, the researcher will report, briefly, the aims of the study, the sample, the data collection and analysis methods used and the findings. In writing proposals for funding, it is usually a requirement that the abstract is written in lay terms. This in itself can be helpful in guiding the researcher towards highly focused research aims and objectives.

Although the abstract is one of the first pages of a research proposal, it is often best written when the proposal is complete. In this way, the abstract more easily becomes a concentrated summary of what the project is about.

Aims and objectives

While the heading of this section is 'aims and objectives', in practice, various terms can be used here. A research project has to be clearly focused, because it is this focus which provides the direction for the research process as the project takes shape. The researcher must know, in advance, what he or she is trying to find out. Most beginning researchers attempt to do too much and the process of narrowing down the focus of interest can be a lengthy and painful one. A useful means of knowing that you have finally identified the *exact* focus for a study is when you can state it in one sentence. For example, the beginning researcher might say, when asked what his or her project is about: 'I want to look at the things students think about reflection and reflective practice. I want to know what their problems with it are and how it affects their clinical practice. I also want to hear about their teachers' experiences of teaching reflective practice and see if they feel that it makes a difference to clinical practice'. After discussion with a research supervisor and a reading of the literature, the answer to the question: 'What is your project about?' might be: 'It is a descriptive study of student midwives' attitudes towards reflective practice'.

Having identified exactly what the project is about, the researcher will write either a set of aims and objectives for the project *or* a number of research questions. Aims are broad, general statements about what the research will be about, while objectives are smaller statements about the actions to be taken. Thus, an aim might be to 'Identify the attitudes of student midwives towards reflective practice', while two objectives might be to '(1) identify an appropriate, convenience sample of student midwives; (2) use a validated instrument to identify student midwives' attitudes towards reflective practice'.

A research question is not dissimilar to a research aim but the focus of the research is demonstrated in a question. For example, 'What are some student midwives' attitudes towards reflective practice?'

In the case of quantitative studies, a hypothesis will be stated – a very specific statement that is to be tested by the research and found to be either 'supported' or 'not supported' at the end of the study. Occasionally, the statistical term, null hypothesis, is used to state that something is *not* likely to be the case at the end of the study (e.g., from the pharmacy world, drug 'A' will not be demonstrated as being more effective in the treatment of hypotension than drug 'B'). Hypothesis testing is discussed in more detail in Chapter 14.

A review of the literature

As we shall see, all researchers need to do a thorough search of the literature that has preceded the study. This search of the literature is to find out what previous research has been done, what others have written about on the topic, and to place the present study in context. Research projects do not simply arise out of the blue. They are always linked, closely, to a particular time in history, a particular set of beliefs that are current about a subject and must always be clearly linked to what is already known about the topic in question.

The development of computer software that allows huge databases of research reports and publications to be searched means that most researchers can now undertake *systematic* reviews of the literature. The aim of a systematic review is to attempt to identify almost every paper that relates to the current topic being researched. This is no easy task, even with computerised search engines. The researcher must identify key words in order for the engines to identify appropriate papers. Once a range of papers has been identified, the researcher then needs to filter these down to *exactly* the papers that are relevant to his or her study. Finally, the papers themselves have to be obtained, read, summarised and their reference formally recorded. Searching the literature is covered in detail in Chapter 4.

In reviewing the literature, in this way, the researcher is also required to read critically. What are the limitations of the study report that is being read? What, if any, mistakes were made in the research process? What else needs to be done? Asking these questions can help further focus on the study being undertaken by the researcher who is doing the review. The critical evaluation of research papers is described near the end of this book in Chapter 22.

It is not always necessary for the researcher to design an entirely new project. There is considerable value in undertaking a *replication study*. In such a study, the methods used in a previous study are used again. If the replication is very close to the original piece of research, much can be learned about whether or not the original work was sound and whether or not the findings from the original are still valid or current.

There is a certain hierarchy in the value of papers that are reviewed. The soundest evidence comes from original report papers. After that, in degrees of value, come theoretical papers, which summarise the research and develop theoretical perspectives. A long way behind these two come 'opinion papers'. These are usually short, one-page papers that appear in many healthcare journals and magazines. They may help to illustrate some of the current debates about certain issues but, in the end, usually only reflect the writer's own views. As a result, they are not particularly useful in generating information for a review.

The most thorough researcher also considers the 'grey literature'. This is that literature which is not formally published in journals or books. Examples of the grey literature include documents such as college reports, curriculum documents and handouts. Again, their status may not be very high in the evidence hierarchy but they can help to identify current trends in a particular discipline.

Some reviewers of the literature attempt a type of content analysis of that literature. This is to say that they count the occurrence of certain issues that arise across a spread of papers and then tabulate their findings. Such counting needs to be done carefully and is probably only really valid when a researcher has managed to identify *all* the literature in a given topic.

A systematic review of the literature means being systematic in other ways too. The researcher must set up appropriate and careful systems for managing the literature that they find. He or she must also be careful to record the exact reference to a given piece of work. Such references (e.g. author, date, title of book or paper, publisher of book or paper, page numbers [in the case of a journal paper]) can be stored either in a dedicated, computerised, reference database (such as *End Note* or *Reference Manager*) or can be stored on cards or in a notebook. What is essential is that the researcher is very clear about how to properly cite references, using either the Harvard or Vancouver systems of citation, and is also very careful to record all the details of a reference for further use in writing the research proposal or report. This point cannot be repeated too much: you MUST know how to reference properly. In our experience, many students at various levels in their academic careers have difficulty with the particular aspect of scholarship. It is worth learning to reference very early on in that career.

The sample

A sample is a slice of any given population. For example, we might consider 'the population' to be those who live in London. A 'sample' would be a selected group of those people.

In quantitative research, there are careful means for selecting a *representative* sample: that is to say, a sample that can, statistically, represent the larger population. The findings from such a sample can sometimes be generalised out to that larger population. There are computer programs for generating a *power calculation* which allows the researcher, in quantitative research, to identify the minimum number required in a sample for representativeness, given the size of the total population. Careful selection of a sample, in quantitative research, is essential for identifying the degree to which findings can or cannot be generalised out to the larger population. These issues are discussed further in Chapters 6 and 13

Generally, in qualitative research, three types of sample are routinely used. Researchers may use a convenience sample, a purposive sample or a snowball sample. A convenience sample is one that is made up of people who happen to be available to take part in the research. For example, in a midwifery department, a particular class or group of classes may constitute a convenience sample. A purposive sample is one made up of people who are reasonably likely to be able to offer information or views on a given topic. For example, it would be pointless asking student midwives who had no experience or knowledge of reflective practice for their views of reflective practice, but much more helpful to ask students who did have such experience or knowledge. We could sample specifically for students who had this experience or knowledge, and such a group would be a purposive sample. Surprisingly, if the whole population of students had such experience, no purposive selection of them according to that criterion would be possible. It would not be appropriate to refer to students from this group who eventually participated in the study as a purposive sample simply because they possessed characteristics we would have wished to select for, because the whole population have this characteristic.

A snowball sample is rather different and is usually used, in qualitative research, when interviews are being conducted. Here, the researcher asks the interviewee, at the end of the interview, to recommend someone else that he or she might interview. Thus, in a study of healthcare education, the interviewer may interview a course leader about the economics of such education. After the interview, the researcher may ask the course leader to recommend another person for interview and the interviewee may suggest the local finance officer. Thus, the pattern of sampling 'snowballs'. Clearly, the snowball sample is also a purposive one. Issues around sampling in qualitative and quantitative research are covered in detail in Chapters 7 and 13, respectively.

Measures and materials

Measurement is usually a feature of quantitative research and involves the selection of measures and scales appropriate to accurate examination of the issues to be explored during the study. In qualitative research, although formal measurement is less frequent, the researcher will want to create detailed interview schedules or guidelines for the completion of field notes. There may also be stimulus materials to be shown to participants. For example, focus group interviews sometimes ask participants to comment on such things as the appropriateness of patient information booklets. In all cases, a clear rationale for the use of particular measures and materials should be described.

Data collection

The most common forms of data, from social science and healthcare research, arise in one of two forms: numbers or words. Occasionally, photographs and other forms of data are also collected and the collection of these seems likely to increase in the future as more sophisticated and computerised methods of data storage and analysis become available.

In quantitative research, the data are mostly likely to be numerical. These figures can come from various sources: they may be scores on a questionnaire, arise out of direct counting of things or may come out of other data sets. In qualitative research, data (in the form of words) usually come from transcripts of interviews or from the researchers' field notes.

A short list of data collection methods to be found in social science and healthcare research might include, at least, the following:

Data collection approaches

- Direct, non-participative, observation by the researcher
- Participative observation (observation made while the researcher is working alongside other people)
- Questionnaires and scales
- Interviews
- Field notes
- Focus groups (or group interviews)
- Historical review of documents
- Meta-analysis of findings from other studies

You will see that no research *designs* are given here. We have not mentioned, for example, ethnography, randomised controlled trials or systematic reviews. This is because designs are basically approaches to organising the way in which data are collected. So, for example, a randomised controlled trial could involve direct observation and the use of scales.

Procedure

Strictly speaking, the procedure is not necessarily data collection, but refers more generally to everything you, as a researcher, do with a research participant. This includes, for example, initial meetings with potential participants to recruit them into the study, gaining consent from them, communicating with them to inform them further about the study, and so on. However, in healthcare research, the idea of a procedure commonly carries the sense of some intervention with participants. Most often these are clinical interventions with patients (e.g., the initiation by physiotherapists of a group class in balance for older patients admitted to hospital following a fall), but quite possibly interventions with staff (comparison of two different initiatives to encourage evidence-based practice) or healthy volunteers (comparison of two methods of presenting information on which to base informed consent to enter a research study).

Data analysis

Although much more is discussed about the analysis of data in other chapters of this book, two broad approaches can be noted here. Numerical data are normally summarised and presented in the form of percentages of responses within the sample. If the correct form of sampling has been used, *inferential statistics* may also be used with these summarised data to identify the degree to which it is safe or not safe to generalise the findings out to the larger population. Perhaps the most widely used computer program for handling numerical data, in social science and healthcare research is *SPSS* (Statistical Package for the Social Sciences).

Textual data are normally content analysed in some way. In this case, transcripts of interviews, group interviews or other written material are summarised under a range of headings and subheadings. As we shall see, there are various approaches to tackling the task of identifying these headings and subheadings. Various computer programs exist for managing qualitative, textual data (e.g., *Atlas ti and The Ethnograph*). It should be noted, however, that whilst a numerical package such as *SPSS* analyses numerical data, a textual data package such as *Atlas ti*, does not. Qualitative data management programs do not *analyse* data they merely assist the researcher in that process. By the same token, statistical packages such as *SPSS* cannot decide for the researcher which test is to be used on the data. The package merely assists by running that test.

Ethical issues

Various ethical issues arise in almost all social science and healthcare research. For example, is the study in question worth doing? Is it likely to do harm to anyone who takes part in the study? Are the methods used likely to help the researcher to achieve his or her aims or answer his or her question? These questions have to be answered: poor or dangerous research is worse than no research at all. Most hospitals and other healthcare-related institutions have their own research ethics committees, to which full research proposals must be submitted and approved – before the research is started. In the UK, there are Local Research Ethics Committees, comprising of medical and healthcare staff and lay members, who consider all larger research proposals. NHS Trusts and universities are now insisting that *all* research that involves people (staff or patients) must be subject to formal ethical approval before a study is begun.

Financial issues

All research that is done in a place of work, involves the spending of money. It is good practice (a) to formally identify the cost of a particular project and (b) to seek approval for the funding of that project. Financial considerations that need to be made include the cost of staff time, the cost of the use of equipment (and, sometimes, the cost of the equipment itself), stationary and photocopying costs, postage and secretarial costs, the cost of any software required for data analysis, travel and related costs. Many colleges and universities have departments which will help provide an accurate costing for a proposed project. If this is available, it is probably best to have such a department work out costs: they will have a better understanding of, in particular, staff costs than the average researcher.

If a study is being submitted for a grant or other sort of funding, the grant-awarding or funding body will insist on a fully worked out costing of the project. Again, this is where a university department that exists to cost projects can be very useful.

Writing the report

Generally, there are two approaches to the writing of a research report. One is to begin the write up at the start of the project and continue to write it throughout the life of the project. The second is to write up the project after the findings have been identified. There is much to commend the former approach. Most sections of a research report reflect the order in which research activities are carried out, so it makes sense to write down what happens in each of the research stages as they happen. The one exception to this is the review of the literature. This is likely to continue throughout the life of the research. One of the last tasks, in any research project, should be to make a final check of the available literature. Most researchers, despite this, have been saddened to find that, immediately after finishing their study, two or three important papers suddenly appear in print!

Most research reports, in their ordering, reflect the stages of the research process as reflected in this chapter. Thus, after an initial introduction, the report will identify the aims and objectives of the study (or the hypothesis or research question). It will then identify the sample and explain how it was derived. The following sections will describe the data collection methods and data analysis methods used. Another section will report the findings of the study. The final section will usually be a discussion of the findings, with the implications of the study being drawn out. There is some debate as to whether such a section should or should not identify the strengths and weaknesses of the study.

Those in favour of reporting strengths and weaknesses might argue that this is a means of evaluating what has been done. No research project is perfect and we can all identify things that went wrong or issues that had not been anticipated. Those who propose not reporting strengths and weaknesses might argue that a given study should stand on its own merits. Presumably, the researcher did the best job that he or she could do and, also, should have been able to anticipate or put right any errors that became apparent. A cynical view might also be that no researcher is going to evaluate the negative points of his or her study to the point where such critical commentary undermines the project.

Publishing the findings

Research is not finished until the study is published. This is the final stage of the research process, or, if we regard that process as cyclical, the starting point for the generation of further research questions, both by the researchers and by those who read their reports of their work. Most researchers aim at publishing their findings in a double-blind refereed journal (e.g., in *Occupational Therapy International*, *Journal of Clinical Nursing*, *British Medical Journal*, *British Journal of Clinical Psychology*). That is to say that their work is considered, anonymously, by at least two referees, who normally are the researcher's peers in the field. These reviewers' judgements are involved in deciding whether a research report is published or not. Some researchers publish shortened versions of their work in more frequently published, professional and popular journals (e.g., in nursing, this might be in the *Nursing Times*, whilst in radiography, *Radiography* is a journal which has a mass readership amongst radiographers, but still maintains a considerable academic profile, which is reflected in the depth of many of its papers).

The journal paper is different from a full research report. Obviously, it is shorter than the full report and many of the initial sections (such as the literature review and methods sections) need to be cut, considerably. Enough must be left, however, to convince the reader that what has been done is sound and appropriate. The bulk of the paper will normally be about the findings of the study.

It cannot be assumed that writing a paper for a 'popular' journal is easier than writing one for an academic journal. The two styles are different. While the academic journal paper is likely to be heavily referenced, the paper for the popular journal is likely to be much more journalistic in style – with the emphasis on short sentences and short paragraphs. Such a style of writing takes practice.

Occasionally, researchers publish their findings in the form of a book (having first published an initial report in a journal). There is a limited market for book-length research reports and a researcher must first obtain a contract from a publisher. This process is not dissimilar to the process of applying for ethical approval. The researcher must first draw up a book proposal – and most publishers can offer examples of these and even pro formas. The book may be quite different from the original research report, with the emphasis very much on the findings of the study. The advantage of writing a book about a research project is that it can free the researcher from (a) the restraints of the 'academic style' and (b) of never making an unsupported claim. A book often allows the researcher to be more discursive and to develop his or her ideas a little (or a lot) further. The decision about where to publish should be informed by ideas about the likely target audience

Timetable

Finally, as with all other projects, the researcher must work to a timetable. Time limits are often imposed by either courses or by funding bodies. Few research projects are completely open-ended and, even if they are, it is always useful to plan the timing of each stage of a project carefully. The research process for any given study must be completed within that time limit.

It is useful to 'work backwards' from the point at which a project has to be completed. Thus, dates can be plotted, in a diary, for each of the processes that have to be completed. In a complicated or large project, it may be useful to use a computerised project planning program, such as *Project*. This allows the researcher to identify, very carefully, how one 'piece of time' affects others. It can also demonstrate how slippage, in one area of the project, is likely to affect other areas. However, such programs are, themselves, quite complicated and most research projects can be managed with a diary and a written-out timetable.

Alongside this form of project planning, it is useful if the researcher keeps a running diary of what happens during the project. A suitable notebook can be used for this, with one page of each two-page section being used to record a stream of events and the other page of each two-page section being used for random notes or theories. The diary thus becomes a log of the whole research project and is a useful aid when writing up the final report.

Other issues

Research involves working through a range of stages and developing a range of skills. Once some of these skills are learned, research need not be difficult to do. However, it is important, in all types of research, to be methodical and honest. Things go wrong. It is important to be able to stop, when they do, make the appropriate corrections, and move on. It is also important to report these errors and mistakes when they occur.

Outside of the obvious skills of knowing 'what to do' to do research, other skills also come into play. The researcher must also be a writer. He or she must not only write a report of what has happened but also be able to write for journals or, as a student, for the completion of assignments. Interpersonal skills are often involved in healthcare research, too. The researcher is likely to have to develop interviewing skills, be able to gain the confidence of his or her respondents and have the diplomatic skills needed to gain access to a sample.

In evidence-based healthcare, research offers most of the evidence. We should neither be frightened of it nor too accepting of it. It is important to develop 'research-mindedness'. That is to say that we should strive, at all times, to ask the question: 'what evidence is there for this?' And to be prepared to seek out such evidence, if it exists. Research-mindedness, then, involves a certain critical response to our work and even to everyday life. Alongside all this, we should try to develop a thorough understanding of the main approaches to research, so that we are able to evaluate the research that we read. Not all research is of equal quality. Despite the checks that are in place to attempt to ensure that only 'good' research gets published, they are not always successful. We all need to develop what the novelist, Ernest Hemingway, called a 'shockproof crap detector'. We need to be able to make reasoned decisions about the relative quality and applicability of a piece of research to our own work. Evidence-based healthcare, then, essentially means *research*-based healthcare.

Organising your own research

There is a riddle, in the form a question, in Southeast Asia and it is this: 'How do you eat an elephant?' The answer is 'a bit at a time'. And so it is with research. At first sight, undertaking any sort of research project can seem a daunting task. The point is to organise it into small, feasible sections.

The primary act in organising your research is to prepare a proposal. A research proposal is a statement of intent: it tells the reader (and the researcher) what is likely to happen during the course of the project. While proposals can be changed (and sometimes circumstances mean that they have to be) it is always best if the proposal can be as accurate and as clear a declaration as possible.

Anyone supervising research will require a proposal from the researcher, as will ethics committees and any boards responsible for approving research. Just as importantly, a good research proposal will act as the map of the research project. It is not simply an exercise in thinking but also a definite plan of action.

It follows from this that it is useful to organise the rest of your project in terms of the research process described above. It logically flows, from the proposal, that a full review of the literature is the second phase of the undertaking, followed by sample selection, access to that sample, measurement selection, data collection and analysis and writing a report. In some cases, these activities will overlap. In particular, the business of reviewing the literature is one that takes place throughout the project: new papers and other texts are being published every week and it is important to keep up to date with these.

Report writing is another activity that can be started almost immediately. A good plan is to use the research process headings to organise your report. If you consider any published research report you will notice that it is organised along these lines. Thus, the chapters of a research report would normally be as follows:

Organisation of the research report

- Abstract
- Introduction
- Aims and objectives
- Sample
- Measures and materials
- Data collection methods
- Data analysis methods
- Ethical issues
- Findings
- Discussion and conclusions
- References

It is useful to open up a new folder, on your computer for your project and open a new file, with the above headings forming their names. It is not necessary to write your report in a linear way (from start to finish) but, instead, return to your files at different times and update them. You may, for example, write the aims and objectives section fairly early on – borrowing from your proposal. You may choose to write the introduction only when you have finished the project. Similarly, the abstract will undoubtedly be the last thing you write.

It is good practice to write every day, if you can. Likewise, all the rules of good writing apply to a research report: you should write simple and clear, using short sentences and short paragraphs. Write to express yourself and not to impress other people. The research report is your report to the rest of the world: you must be honest and clear in writing it. The usual guidance given is that you should write your methods out to the point where another person could easily replicate your studies – and this is good advice. If your work is to be assessed as part of a diploma, degree or higher degree, it is essential that those marking it know exactly what you have done. Report writing is mentioned in more detail in Chapter 23.

Exercise

This is the longest exercise in this book. Without reading any further in this book, consider each phase in the research process and relate it to your own proposed research project, constructing a *Research Log* of your ideas. (If you do not already have a project in mind, it is worthwhile spending a few minutes now generating a possible idea from your clinical practice which might make a good research topic.)

To do this, you should work through each heading in this chapter and ask yourself what it means *practically* for your research idea. For example, how will you collect the data?

Keep your *Research Log* close to you as you read this book. Each time you come to relevant material later in the book, return to this exercise and examine the relevant section, modifying it in light of what you have subsequently learned. For example, when you read the chapters on sampling, return to the *Sample* section in your *Research Log*, and note down any necessary changes from what you originally thought.

A pro forma to help you construct this log is given at the end of this book as Appendix 1, and there are several pages, so you can write straight into this book if you want. For those of you who do not like to do that, you are welcome to photocopy the appendix. You may prefer to copy the headings into a computer. Where whole chapters are devoted to particular aspects of organising the research, these chapters are noted on the pro forma.

Good luck with your log. One bonus in using it is that it is similar in structure to the research proposals required by many courses, funding bodies and ethics committees, so you can, for example, start using it right away to help you with a future research assignment.

Further reading

Bell, J. (2005) *Doing Your Research Project: A Guide for First-Time Researchers in Education, Health and Social Sciences.* Milton Keynes: Open University Press.

Bowling, A. (2002) *Research Methods in Health: Investigating Health and Health Services.* Milton Keynes: Open University Press.

Burnard, P. (2004) *Writing Skills in Health Care.* Gloucester: Stanley Thornes.

Crotty, M. (1998) *The Foundations of Social Research: Meaning and Perspective in the Research Process.* London: Sage.

Gray, A. (2003) *Research Practice for Cultural Studies.* London: Sage.

Choosing Methodological Approaches

Key points

- Researchers tend to associate inductive reasoning with qualitative research and theory building, and deductive reasoning
  with quantitative research and theory testing.
- Quantitative approaches emphasise cause–effect relationships
  and prediction.
- Qualitative approaches emphasise exploration.
- Researchers should examine the goals of their research when
  choosing methodological approaches.
- Consider qualitative approaches first for studies of experience
  individuals, research with excluded and hard to reach groups
  and pilot studies.
- Consider quantitative approaches first for epidemiological
  studies of large groups and treatment comparison studies.

Introduction

The choice of a general methodological approach is informed by many
different issues, some subjective, some theoretical and some practical. For example, it used to be common, for undergraduate and

---

Research for Evidence-Based Practice in Healthcare, Second edition, by Robert Newell and Philip Burnard
© 2011 Robert Newell and Philip Burnard

pre-registration dissertations, and even up to PhD level, to encourage students to undertake studies using whatever methods most interested them. Intuitively, this seems a good course of action, because we want students to complete their projects, and have good reason to believe that they will be more likely to complete undertakings which involve them in things they are interested in. However, the counterargument is that this kind of supposed freedom has too many negative consequences to make it advisable. First, we might hope that student research will be useful to others as well as to the student, and following one's methodological preferences in an unfettered way may lead to the undertaking of projects which lend themselves to a particular methodological approach, rather than to those of obvious benefit to patients. Moreover, if a student is sponsored by their employer, the employer will very likely have views as to the sort of project they would like to see carried out. This may not fit with student methodological preferences. Equally, there is the possibility that methodological preference may result in a researcher making a research question fit with a particular approach, regardless of whether that approach is appropriate (see the discussion of qualitative and quantitative approaches).

Perhaps most important, however, is the view of science that the 'personal preference' approach to methodological choice supports. This is the view that science is an individual, personal activity. Whilst this is certainly true in the sense that considerable personal skill and commitment are involved, science is mostly (and, arguably, most importantly) a social activity. It is carried out by groups of people, reviewed by and communicated to groups of people, and, at least in health research, undertaken for the good of society. In our view, any teaching of research which does not emphasise that gives at best a partial view of the nature of the research endeavour. Accordingly, we advise that the only reasonable rationale for deciding on a methodological approach is on the basis of its fitness for purpose.

When is a methodological approach fit for purpose?

Fitness for purpose requires that something does the job it is intended for. In research terms, this implies a number of things. First, the methodological approach must be capable, in principle, of answering the question it seeks to answer. Second, it must be practicable. Third, it must be within the expertise of the researcher. More broadly, there must, as we saw in the previous chapter, be a question which is worth answering (because it has not been adequately answered before and will tell us something of value).

Two different approaches to knowledge

Writers about *epistemology* (the study of the nature of knowledge) like to talk about deductive and inductive approaches to knowledge as representing two broad approaches to its generation. Although there has been debate about whether these two terms are truly separate, the distinction is certainly current in science. Basically, deductive investigation is said to proceed from a general standpoint (such as a known theory) and examine specific instances which confirm or disconfirm that general view. By contrast, inductive investigation is supposed to involve starting with specific instances and deriving a general conclusion from them. These are sometimes described as top-down and bottom-up approaches, respectively.

For example, investigating the general concept of habituation (the tendency to cease to respond to repeatedly presented stimuli) by conducting a series of experiments in which students were submitted to sudden, loud noises, and recording variations in their heart rates on successive presentations is an example of deductive research. Asking students about their experiences of such loud noises and seeking to find commonalities in their responses which might lead us to theorise about the nature of that common experience is inductive.

As we noted above, there is debate about the independence of these forms of inquiry. For example, the philosopher John Stuart Mill, in his discussion of deduction, regards induction as part of the process. Part of the issue here is that different writers use these terms in slightly different ways, and this has affected the way in which we talk about the distinction between induction and deduction. A detailed discussion of the relationship between deductive and inductive reasoning is beyond the scope of this book. However, many people are familiar with the deductions of Sherlock Holmes, and a very readable and enjoyable account of inductive and deductive reasoning using Holmes as an example is available at http://www.bun.kyoto-u.ac.jp/~suchii/holmes_1.html.

Different broad methodological approaches and their appropriateness

In research, there has been a tendency to associate inductive reasoning with qualitative research and theory building, and deductive reasoning with quantitative research and theory testing. However, this is not a hard and fast rule. For example, a small survey might possibly be a reasonable way of generating ideas which would then lead to some general hypotheses about the world which would be tested in larger studies. Here, a quantitative method is proceeding from the specific to the general. Likewise, many qualitative studies end up by referring back to existing theories, although whether they could justifiably be called tests of such theories is another matter. Finally, mixed methods studies seek to combine qualitative and quantitative approaches, but do not necessarily combine theory building and theory testing.

Nevertheless, the broad alignment of qualitative research with inductive reasoning and quantitative with deductive is probably a useful rule of thumb. For the researcher, it may be most useful to combine such ideas with an examination of the researcher's goals for the project. These will almost always be framed as research questions. Looked at in this way, our grounds for choosing qualitative versus quantitative methods are clearer. Broadly speaking, qualitative methods are better employed at the beginning of the life of a research question, when little is known about the subject. You can see that this is tied to the idea of theory building. By its nature, a problem we know little about is often unlikely to be associated with major existing theories. However, one thing which the novice should beware of is assuming that this is the case. For example, imagine we are examining the information needs of people who have experienced surgery which has caused a change in their facial appearance. As it happens, there is comparatively little research into this area. Nevertheless, there are any number of theories which are relevant and might bear testing in this group. We do not necessarily have to assume that a new series of qualitative studies using inductive methods is necessary to build new theory. However, it may still be the case that we will want to do some initial qualitative work to get an idea of these people's experiences.

Quantitative approaches, by contrast, are best used when quite a lot is known about a topic area. Often, quantitative approaches, particularly treatment comparisons, come at a stage when a research question has been under examination for some considerable time, and is well integrated with a particular theory. Indeed, there may actually be competing accounts of what factors impact on the question, and these may be associated with different theories. Quantitative approaches attempt to tease out cause–effect relationships and establish predictive models associated with established theories, often allowing us to judge between the usefulness of competing models and theories. As with qualitative research, however, this is not always the way in which quantitative methods are used. Even in the absence of any theory, it would be perfectly possible to compare different approaches to care using, for example, a randomised controlled trial (RCT), to see which worked best for patients. The rationale for so doing might have no theory attached to it, but be driven simply by having observed these two different practices in the clinical setting. Given that a good deal of healthcare is based on tradition, this is quite likely, and finding evidence to support one practice rather than another can validly occur in the absence of any underlying theory.

Given that the associations between inductive reasoning and qualitative methods and between deductive reasoning and quantitative methods are not mutually exclusive, what other guidelines might we use to decide the general appropriateness of the two approaches? One distinction we have already met is the one based on the maturity of the research question. By maturity, we mean the amount of investigation it has received. As we noted, qualitative methods are better suited early in this process, and quantitative ones later. Associated with this notion are the ideas of exploration, explanation and prediction. Early in the life of a research question, much of the work is exploratory, and qualitative work is, arguably, better at this type of activity, because it examines individual cases in great detail. Some level of explanation of the characteristics is then possible, but that explanation is best pursued in further quantitative studies, because part of the notion of explanation is that it should hold good in general, not just in relation to the specific sample being studied. Qualitative and quantitative approaches make different suppositions about explanation and generalisation, and these are explored in the relevant sections of this book.

However, by and large, quantitative research places more emphasis on the generalisation of results to large populations. Moreover, this type of research is often concerned with the idea of the prediction of behaviour. For example, when we examine the action of a drug in a sample of patients we actually want to be able to predict how it will behave, in general, in patients in the future. Similarly, if we are looking at a healthcare intervention such as reassurance, we want to know, in broad terms, how patients will respond to it in the future.

This emphasis on prediction led to a reaction against quantitative methods amongst nurses in particular, but also other groups of HCPs, because it was felt that such an emphasis ran contrary to the view of healthcare practice as an individualised, patient-centred activity. Happily, much of this debate has now subsided, as most doctors and other healthcare professionals now recognise the complementary strengths of individualised care planning and effective general interventions which can be tailored to individuals. In the same way, at their best, qualitative and quantitative approaches can go hand in hand. Without the generalisability of quantitative research, we would have no rationale for using a treatment which had proved useful with one patient on another, but without qualitative research, we would often never have discovered the treatment to begin with.

One factor which can drive our decisions about research methodology is this understanding of the difference between individual and general experiences. This distinction precisely characterises the major difference between qualitative and quantitative methods. Researchers wishing to investigate personal experiences in detail will be most likely to find a qualitative approach fulfils their needs best, as this type of research allows the flexibility to work in depth with a few respondents and help them to give detailed accounts of their experiences. By contrast, researchers who are interested in drawing conclusions about what large groups of people experience will typically use quantitative approaches. Here, detail and, to a marked extent, flexibility, are sacrificed in order to allow this general picture to emerge. There has to be this trade-off for two reasons. First, if we want to know what groups of people experience, we usually have to research large numbers, and if we do this, we do not have the resource to get a great amount of detail from each respondent and then analyse it. Second, we will want to gather the data in a specified, systematised (usually, numerical) format, because this will allow us to examine the data in a way which permits us to draw conclusions about the population as a whole (see Chapter 5).

What sorts of questions for what general approaches?

Having explored the general rationale behind qualitative and quantitative approaches, we will now consider the kinds of specific issues you might use each approach to investigate. This discussion is by no means exhaustive, and much of it will be amplified in the sections of this book concerned with the two approaches. What we intend here is a series of illustrations which might help you in deciding how research questions might best be tackled.

We suggested that qualitative research was at its best when dealing with the detailed examination of individual experiences, and also noted its role in theory building and exploration. It follows from this that the following sorts of areas are best examined qualitatively, certainly in the first instance:

Patients' and carers' experience of illness and care. Typically, researchers will use unstructured or semi-structured interviews to approach this broad topic area. These allow detailed exploration and the opportunity for the respondent to tell their own story in their own way.

Research with excluded and hard to reach groups. Here, qualitative approaches using interview and observation have several advantages. Apart from allowing detailed exploration, qualitative approaches may be more acceptable to the target groups, as they are, arguably, less formal and more collaborative. Finally, by their nature, these groups have been less frequently researched than others and, in consequence, research from them will benefit from an inductive approach to theory building.

Pilot and feasibility studies. When we are developing a new intervention, we want to know as much as possible about precisely how it is being carried out and the reaction of patients. There may well be an element of quantitative analysis in such studies, but the detailed observation and conversational questioning familiar to qualitative researchers has a lot to offer in describing the exact circumstances which may influence effectiveness and acceptability of an intervention. Additionally, such approaches can tell us about potential methodological problems in mounting a treatment study.

Quantitative approaches, by contrast, are best at examining general trends in large groups:

Patients' and carers' experience of illness and care. The type of research appropriate here will probably be by means of surveys, and will almost always follow on from a qualitative study. The difference between qualitative and quantitative examinations of experiences is essentially that approaches like surveys give a broad-brush picture of groups of people's experiences, rather than those of individuals.

Epidemiological studies. These studies are essentially survey approaches, possibly using elements of observation. Their aim is to identify trends in populations with regard to the behaviour (usually, an illness or response to it) under examination. Both the survey and observational components will be carried out using strict sampling protocols and standardised measurement procedures to ensure that accurate rates emerge which are generalisable to the whole population.

Treatment comparison studies. Typically, the researcher will be keen to ensure no bias which might alter apparent treatment effects intrudes into these studies. Accordingly, quantitative researchers have developed a series of different research designs which attempt to reduce bias so that the relationship between treatment and outcome is relatively clear. Probably the most well known and methodologically adequate of these (but also the most difficult to mount) is the RCT, in which patients are randomly allocated to receive one or another treatment. In some situations, it is possible to offer the treatment in such a way that neither the patient nor the clinician knows who is receiving which treatment. In situations where RCTs are not possible, other designs such as non-randomised designs and before–after designs may be used. The same standardised measurement and treatment delivery are used as in RCTs, but there is greater opportunity for bias.

Do we need to do research at all?

All research is hard to carry out. Apart from methodological problems, there are difficulties with organising treatments across different sites, recruiting respondents, ensuring the safety of respondents, ensuring adequate expertise to analyse the data appropriately. For this reason, it is important to be clear that a piece of research actually needs carrying out. We can see two main reasons for doing a piece of healthcare research: it addresses an important question; it responds to a gap in the literature. In the first instance, we will agree that the question is important if it has consequences for our understanding of health and illness and if it is likely to lead to improvement in the delivery of care. In the second case, we will want to be sure that an issue has not been examined before, or has not been examined adequately. The principal way of establishing this is via review of the existing literature. This consists of two parts: searching and appraising. We examine these issues in Chapters 4 and 22, respectively.

Review questions

Is science a personal or a social activity (or somewhere in between)? What are the implications of our answers to this for selection of a research method?

What *approaches* to knowledge are generally associated with qualitative and quantitative research?

What types of *question* are best answered by qualitative or quantitative research?

Exercise

What is the first issue about your own clinical practice which comes to your mind as needing investigation? Ask yourself the following questions about it:

What gaps are there in our knowledge of this issue?
What kind of a question might I ask to address some of these gaps?
What sort of method might be useful to ask this question?

Further reading

Holloway, I. and Wheeler, S. (1996) *Qualitative Research for Nurses*. Oxford: Blackwell Science.

Hoskins, C. and Mariano, C. (2004) *Research in Nursing and Health: Understanding and Using Quantitative and Qualitative Methods*. New York: Springer.

Thompson, D. and Martin, C. (2001) *Design and Analysis of Clinical Nursing Research Studies*. London: Routledge.

Website

http://www.fortunecity.com/greenfield/grizzly/432/rra2.htm

Searching the Literature

Key points

- Literature searches are done primarily to ensure awareness of a field of research.
- Systematic reviews examine the literature using systematised and transparent criteria.
- A search strategy consists of the research question, its components, sources of information, search terms, retrieval and inclusion criteria and available resources.
- Sensitivity (recall) refers to comprehensivity of a search strategy.
- Specificity (precision) refers to relevance of a search strategy.
- The scope of a search is determined by its search strategy.

Introduction

In Chapter 3, we examined different broad approaches to undertaking research, but also noted that there are only specific circumstances when we would want to do any research at all. One of these was that we should want to be sure that the issue we want to research had not, in fact, been adequately explored before. There are two steps in

Research for Evidence-Based Practice in Healthcare, Second edition, by Robert Newell and Philip Burnard
© 2011 Robert Newell and Philip Burnard

determining this: searching the existing literature to find out whether any work has been done on our topic; critically evaluating (appraising) any literature that does exist to arrive at a judgement as to whether it is good enough, or relevant enough to our topic, to allow us to be confident that further research is not required by us. If work already exists, and it is high-quality, relevant work, we can proceed to a consideration of how to implement that work in practice, rather than having to do primary research.

In this chapter, we explore how to search the literature. We will begin with a description of the *systematic review*, the gold standard in terms of literature reviews, and occasions when it might or might not be possible for you to undertake such a review. The rest of the chapter will focus on practical issues of how to conduct the search for a literature review. Appraising the literature is covered in Chapter 22.

Purpose of literature searches

The first goal of a literature search is to ensure that you are aware of other research in your field. This is important because it is wasteful of resources and probably unethical to carry out research into a topic which has already been adequately explored. If you do not know what is out there, you cannot appropriately appraise it in order to discover whether further research is necessary. Even if you are not considering carrying out primary research, but simply want to discover what is best practice in order to implement it in your clinical area (itself no easy task), an adequate search is a necessary first step. Just as you cannot reasonably decide whether to carry out research in a particular field of practice, likewise, you cannot change practice on the basis of published research without comprehensive literature searching. Once again, this is because adequate appraisal is only possible after adequate search and retrieval. If our search strategy was inadequate and led us to miss important work, we might erroneously assume there was inadequate evidence to implement a particular change in practice. Conversely, a poor search might lead us to uncover research which, in itself, would lead us to implement its findings, but might miss important further work or critique which refuted the findings of this research. Thus, familiarity with the literature is a prerequisite of all aspects of research and its implementation.

Surprisingly, this goal of familiarity, whilst obvious, is not as easily achieved as might be expected. In the past, clinicians and researchers familiar with a particular area have assumed that they knew where the important literature was to be found and, as a result, have followed quite idiosyncratic search methods. With the advent of computer databases of publications, this problem has become even more acute, since the amount of information available became greater without being matched by equal sophistication in literature searching ability. For the student, the problem is even more daunting. Students are, quite reasonably, novices in their area of clinical practice and, often, in academic activity. Most experienced clinical practitioners and academics are familiar with students reporting they have been unable to find references for their essays and suggesting that the evidence does not exist. Unfortunately, the response has often been to blame the student for this mistaken impression, rather than offering systematic advice on what to do about it. This is a shame, because that advice is actually very simple: be clear about what you want to find out about and look in as many places as possible! Unlike a lot of simple advice, however, this particular piece of advice is reasonably easy to follow, because the advent of the systematic review has resulted in clear guidelines as to how to go about searching literature in such a way as to maximise the likelihood of finding relevant material and minimise the chances of being snowed under by references which are irrelevant.

Systematic reviews

A systematic review is a process of identifying the aim of a literature review, then carrying out the search and appraisal of that literature according to set, transparent criteria which are auditable and repeatable by others.

Centre for Reviews and Dissemination (CRD) definition of a systematic review

The systematic review is a 'scientific tool which can be used to summarise, appraise, and communicate the results and implications of otherwise unmanageable quantities of research'. (NHS Centre for Reviews & Dissemination, 2001)

The systematic review strives to be comprehensive and to include all the relevant studies. This provides an overview of the field under examination. Moreover, because the process whereby the review has been conducted is available to the scrutiny of the reader, we can ourselves appraise the process by which the literature has been searched and appraised. The ability to do this is critical to our ability to judge the adequacy of the overview provided in the systematic review.

Two major institutions are currently involved in carrying out systematic reviews in health – the Centre for Reviews and Dissemination (CRD) and the Cochrane Collaboration. Their websites are given at the end of this chapter, and they make synopses of their findings available over the internet, as well as via paper publication. The undertaking of a systematic review is a considerable one, and, in the case of the Cochrane Collaboration, not a time limited one. Members of a Cochrane review group undertake to update their reviews on a frequent and regular basis. The extent of the work in conducting a systematic review is such that research funders regularly offer funding of thousands of pounds for reviews of topics of interest to them. Looking for the existence of a CRD or Cochrane Collaboration review is, therefore, the first step in any literature search, because the busy clinician may well find that this painstaking work has largely or entirely been done for them.

Search process

From the previous paragraph, it seems as if conducting a systematic review is beyond the scope of any single individual, and certainly beyond the scope of a lone student or clinician. However, this is not always the case. In some situations, a field of work is so well defined or so under-developed that a comprehensive review is possible even with limited resources of finance, personnel and time. In recognition of this, many undergraduate courses in nursing involve a dissertation module which consists of a systematic review of a well-defined clinical topic. Even where conducting a systematic review is beyond the resources of an individual (as in many student projects), using the principles involved is still a valuable way of structuring a literature search in order to ensure the maximum comprehensivity and relevance under the circumstances. This chapter is not a guide to systematic reviewing, but shows how the principles can be applied to searching the literature.

Designing a search strategy

The aim of a search is to gain as comprehensive and relevant a picture of the literature as possible. The research strategy determines how far this aim will be met and involves a considerable number of personal choices by the reviewer. Often, the design of this strategy will be done in collaboration with a librarian (usually, a subject specialist in health matters). The reviewer typically brings specialist knowledge of the clinical area, whilst the librarian brings expertise in understanding the organisation of text material and how it is best retrieved. The notions of comprehensivity and relevance are often referred to by systematic reviews as *sensitivity* or *recall* and *specificity* or *precision*, respectively. These notions are similar to the same concepts in other areas of research (e.g., screening for illness risk factors) and are basic to the generation of a search strategy. Sensitivity refers to the number of relevant studies returned by a search strategy expressed as a percentage of the number of such relevant studies that actually exist in the literature, whilst specificity is the number of relevant studies as a proportion of the sum of relevant and irrelevant studies which exist. The development of a strategy which appropriately balances these two issues is largely a process of trial and error, and the main point to be grasped is that it is unwise to stop after a single search. It is likely to be either too sensitive (swamping the reviewer with irrelevant material) or too specific (resulting in the situation we mentioned above), where the review mistakenly supposes that little literature exists. The best advice we can give is to conduct several searches and see what they yield, then reflect on what shortcomings in the search strategy have led to the differing findings. This kind of reflection is best done in collaboration with others who are also familiar with the clinical area.

Components of a search strategy

Several factors contribute to the sensitivity and specificity of a search and, therefore, to the amount and relevance of the material which will be unearthed. These factors are listed in Figure 4.1. Each one is discussed below with regard to its impact on search strategy. For a comprehensive guide to the conduct of reviews, see CRD Report 4, available for the CRD website (address at the end of this chapter).

The research question and its components (referred to as 'facets' in the CRD report) are the first step in defining the scope of the review. For example, consider the likely difference in asking the four questions in Figure 4.2.

Simply put: the more specific the question, the more focal the resulting search. The same thing applies to the search question components. CRD Report 4 describes four possible facets: population, interventions, outcomes and study design. Not all these need be included in every search, and some arise naturally from the research question. In Figure 4.2, there are three different populations and two different interventions, whilst the outcome (benefits) is very generally stated. The question and its explicit facets become more specific as we move from Question 1 to Question 4. Restricting the nature of the outcome and specifying the type of study to be examined (randomised controlled

---

The research question
The question's components
The sources of information
The search terms
The retrieval inclusion criteria
The available resources

Figure 4.1   Factors to consider in designing a search strategy.

1   What benefits, if any, are conferred by complementary therapies in the treatment of cancer?
2   What benefits, if any, are conferred by complementary therapies in the treatment of breast cancer?
3   What benefits, if any, are conferred by acupuncture in the treatment of breast cancer?
4   What benefits, if any, are conferred by acupuncture in the treatment of lymphoedema following surgery for breast cancer?

Figure 4.2   Specificity of search questions.

trials?) will further specify the nature of the question and restrict the search. Specification of question and facets is a powerful way to structure the search, and so should be done sensitively and reflectively, considering the likely consequences of each decision in terms of how it well it fits with your aims and the resulting effects on sensitivity and specificity.

The amount of information which will be gathered is affected by the focus of the review, but also by the breadth of sources of information searched. Searches usually begin with a scrutiny of electronic databases (see Figure 4.3). However, for a comprehensive review, such a search is rarely enough. Lesser-known journals may not be on the databases, whilst *publication bias* may result in only certain types of study being reported. Perhaps the most well known (and potentially important) form of publication bias is the tendency of journals to publish only studies with significant findings, and only original studies (as opposed to replication studies). This tendency is an important source of bias because negative findings are of value, whilst replication studies (particularly failures to replicate findings) are an important check in quantitative research, which is probabilistic in nature. Well-conducted replication studies which do not support the findings of an original study cast doubt on the original findings because they suggest that these originally significant finding may have been the result of a *type I error* (see

MEDLINE
EMBASE
(Both medically oriented databases)
CINAHL
(Database of nursing and allied health papers)
PsycInfo
(Comprehensive psychology database)
CCTR
(Cochrane Controlled Trials Register – contains information not necessarily on MEDLINE or EMBASE)

Figure 4.3   Major health-related databases.

Chapter 20). In order to find such studies, we need to go beyond the results of electronic searches. Typically, this involves hunting down references cited in studies found in electronic searches, including unpublished work, or work which has been published outside the academic arena (so-called 'grey literature' such as internal reports, working papers, theses, newspaper articles). It is also important to search for conference proceedings, where new and emerging work may first be presented. For such new work, research registers such as the national Research Register (https://portal.nihr.ac.uk/Pages/NRRArchive.aspx) is an excellent source, and a comprehensive review will examine this register and similar ones and follow up potentially relevant work in progress by contacting the researchers. In the case of reviews of the effectiveness of drugs and medical appliances and devices, a comprehensive review should involve contacting manufacturers, who have often undertaken research which never finds its way into the academic journals. They may be willing to share their findings with reviewers. Finally, the internet is a vast source of unregulated publication, much of it of dubious quality. It is, nevertheless, a potentially relevant source, at least as a first step in unearthing grey literature and contacting people researching in the same area. Patients and carers can make an important contribution to literature reviews, as they may have considerable experience of searching for materials which relate to their health issues. This expertise can be especially useful in addressing the grey literature.

The final major factor impacting on sensitivity and specificity is the range and character of the search terms employed by the reviewer. In general, a search strategy should use sufficient search terms of sufficient breadth to yield the maximum number of relevant articles ('hits'). Thus, the reviewer identifies search keyword synonyms and variations in spelling, and makes decisions about what combinations of keywords to use in order to limit the search appropriately. Many of the large databases have built-in thesaurus functions to help the reviewer identify synonyms, as well as offering the opportunity to limit the search in a number of ways. Medical subject headings (MeSH) is a frequently used approach to organising a literature search, and for your interest, an informative paper is referenced at the end of this chapter.

Retrieval and inclusion criteria

Having implemented the above phases of the search strategy and found as many apparently relevant studies as possible, you now have to decide whether or not to actually get hold of each paper and if so, whether to include each one in the review. Some of this work can be done at the very beginning of the search. For example, you might decide to search for only qualitative studies, only RCTs or only English language journals. Naturally, you would want some explicit rationale for so doing. However, later on, when you have your list of potential papers to be included, there are still decisions to be made regarding retrieval and inclusion. In terms of retrieval, you may, for example, decide not to retrieve papers where it is clear from the abstract that it is not relevant. If you cannot decide from the abstract, it is best practice to get the paper anyway, and accept the wasted time if it turns out not to be relevant. Regarding inclusion, even after retrieval you may decide to exclude a paper from the review on grounds of relevance or on grounds of quality. In the case of RCTs, for instance, you might wish to exclude studies which were not randomised via distant allocation or which were not *double blinded* (see Chapter 17). The guiding principle for excluding studies is that you have a rationale for the decisions you make, and that this is agreed and recorded before the process begins. You may have to change your decisions in the light of emerging data in the review, but if so, once again, your reasoning should be recorded and be clear to the reader.

Resources

Naturally, the resources available to a single student are much less than those available to a group of professional reviewers, and teachers will certainly take account of this if marking a literature review assignment. Lack of resources is not, however, an academically valid reason for limiting a search. Accordingly, where you read a review paper which offers such a reason for limiting a search, you should read the review in that light. If, for example, a reviewer has not searched grey literature owing to lack of resource, that is potentially a serious criticism of the review, for the reasons suggested above.

Reporting your search

One point we have made several times in this chapter is the need for the search strategy to be transparent. To this end, your literature review should include a detailed description of the search strategy, including all the elements presented in Figure 4.1. In theory, the description should enable readers to repeat your search for themselves. At the very least it allows them to critically appraise in detail the search choices you have made. Even if you do not have the resources to carry out a full-blown systematic review, employing the same kind of approach, as described here, will give a reasonably comprehensive review, and will also help your reader towards an awareness of its strengths and limitations.

Review questions

What is the first step in a literature search and why?
What factors influence the amount of information which will be collected in a search?
What are the advantages and disadvantages of high and low sensitivity and specificity of a search?

Exercise

Look again at the four search questions in the early part of this chapter. Try and make a more specific search question, then, use the headings in Figure 4.1 to devise a search strategy. Now apply the same process to a question of your own.

Reference

NHS Centre for Reviews & Dissemination (2001) *Undertaking Systematic Reviews of Research on Effectiveness: CRD's Guidance for Those Carrying Out or Commissioning Reviews. CRD* Report Number 4, 2nd edn. York: University of York. Available from CRD's website.

Further reading

Hart, C. (2001) *Doing a Literature Search*. London: Sage.

Lowe, H.J. and Barnett, G.O. (1994) Understanding and using the medical subject headings (MeSH) vocabulary to perform literature searches. *JAMA*, 271, 1103–1108.

Websites

http://www.cochrane.org

http://www.york.ac.uk/inst/crd/

Ethics of Healthcare Research

Key points

- Codifications of research ethics date from the Nuremberg Code and the Declaration of Helsinki.
- Autonomy, beneficence, non-maleficence and justice are key principles in research ethics.
- Autonomy refers to an individual's freedom to choose and act.
- Beneficence requires that we maximise good and minimise harm.
- Justice is the maximising of fairness to all.
- Research ethics committees (RECs) exist to interpret these concepts for the protection of research participants and researchers.
- All research should receive ethical scrutiny.
- All National Health Service (NHS)-related research must receive approval from a REC.
- NHS REC approval is centrally organised and standardised.
- All NHS research must receive Research Governance approval from the NHS institution in which it takes place.
- Research Governance approval is locally organised by each institution and there is limited standardisation.

Research for Evidence-Based Practice in Healthcare, Second edition, by Robert Newell and Philip Burnard
© 2011 Robert Newell and Philip Burnard

Introduction

Ethics is basic to healthcare, and so should be basic to healthcare research. We are discussing these issues here in the first section of this book because we hope they will guide you in your dealings with healthcare research. Healthcare ethics has undergone much change in the past few years, partly because of well-publicised cases of the abuse of patients and tissues from deceased patients in pursuit of research goals. As a result, ethical monitoring of health research is stricter than it has ever been. We will consider this monitoring procedure later in this chapter. For the moment, however, we will examine some of the chief concepts of ethics which are particularly relevant to research and which should guide not only the practice of researchers, but also the practice of the knowledgeable consumer of research findings.

Many commentators date key issues in health research ethics to the Nuremberg Code. The ten provisions of this code are reported in full in numerous papers (see end of chapter), but may be summarised as in Figure 5.1. The code provided the basis for the Declaration of Helsinki in 1964, which was subsequently adopted by many countries engaged in health research, including the UK.

Whilst these provisions might seem obvious to us, they arose, as the name suggests, from the atrocities committed by Nazi scientists and others during the Second World War, in the name of research. Whilst we all hope that no event to rival the horrors of the Holocaust will ever happen again, it is instructive to reflect that even today, many innovations in ethics come as the result of our growing understanding of *unethical* behaviour. This is as true of research as of any other aspect of human experience.

The duties outlined in the Nuremberg Code reflect some basic ethical principles which underpin the way in which research proposals are

---

1. Voluntary consent is essential.
2. Study should yield fruitful results for the good of society.
3. Previous results should justify the study.
4. Study should avoid all unnecessary physical and mental suffering and injury.
5. No study should be conducted if it is believed death or disabling injury will occur.
6. The degree of risk should never exceed potential benefit of the study.
7. Participants should be protected against even remote possibilities of injury, disability or death.
8. The study should be conducted only by qualified persons.
9. Participants should be free to withdraw at any time.
10. The person undertaking the study must be prepared to stop the study if a continuation is likely to cause harm.

Figure 5.1 Synopsis of the Nuremberg code.

reviewed for ethical appropriateness. These principles include the notions of autonomy, beneficence, non-maleficence and justice, and these four principles now form the core of much healthcare ethics practice in the UK, principally because of the work of Beauchamp and Childress (2001) in the US and Gillon (2003) in the UK. Autonomy refers to the recognition that people (including research participants) have the right to decide on a particular course of action and follow it. Naturally, in order to do so, a person must have reasonable awareness of the nature of what they are intending to do and its likely consequences. From this notion, it follows that we must offer people adequate information about a study and the opportunity to give or withhold consent. Again, these two ideas are linked, because it is logically impossible to consent to something if you do not have adequate information about it, or if some aspect of it is deliberately concealed from you. Actually, some studies do involve aspects of deception (without which they would be impossible to conduct), but these are few and far between today (two very famous earlier ones are given as further reading at the end of this chapter), and the rules governing the conduct of and consent process for studies involving deception are extremely stringent. Likewise, to preserve autonomy, people must be free from coercion. For example, it is unethical to state or imply that a person's routine treatment might be affected if they refuse to participate in a research programme, to suggest that a member of staff's conditions of employment might be affected, or to suggest that a student's marks in assignments might be affected by participation in research within an educational institution. In the same way, it is often very difficult for patients to refuse requests to participate in research from people charged with their care, because patients may *believe* that these powerful people can influence their care even when this is not, in fact, the case.

In the context of research, beneficence refers to the requirement that the researcher should maximise benefit to participants whilst minimizing harm. The broad rule of thumb is that the chance of benefit should always outweigh the chance of harm. This has given rise, amongst other things, to the situation where completely unproved treatments (of which there are many in medicine and healthcare) cannot be withheld from patients in the absence of very strong arguments to the contrary. The reason for this is somewhat obscure. After all, if some treatment has no evidence behind it, what possible objection could there to for withholding it? In fact, there are at least a couple. First, it is argued, quite rightly, that lack of evidence of effectiveness is not evidence of lack of effectiveness, and there is a fair case for saying that a treatment which has been in use for many years might confer some benefit, even if we have yet to amass the evidence for that benefit. Proponents of evidence-based practice are, paradoxically, often very keen to make this point in reporting the findings of systematic reviews. Balanced against this, however, we might take the commonsense view that (a) interventions often survive because of the vested interests of powerful people even if ineffective and unpopular, and (b) if a treatment that had been in use for many years was effective, one would have expected to find evidence of that effectiveness by now. We leave it to you to judge between these competing arguments. The second argument against the withholding of unproven treatments is, we feel, less contentious. If a patient knew that a treatment was being withheld, they might suffer *psychological* damage, on the basis that they were aware that it had been offered in the past and that some people, rightly or wrongly, believed it was effective or that they had received benefit from it. Moreover, because there are clear associations between psychological distress and recovery from illness, this distress might indeed affect their physical response and do them harm. Of course, offering unproven treatments is not in any obvious way a major act of beneficence, either in the research context or any other. Moreover, offering such a treatment infringes a person's autonomy by compromising their ability to give informed consent, unless it is made completely clear to them that the treatment offered is of no proven value.

Four principles of healthcare ethics

Autonomy – respect people's right to exercise their freedom
Beneficence – do good when possible
Non-maleficence – avoid doing harm
Justice – treat people fairly

Whilst it is hard to say which of the four principles mentioned here is pre-eminent, non-maleficence (the avoidance of doing harm or the risk of doing harm), might be a good candidate (although at least one famous medical ethicist has argued otherwise (Gillon, 2003)). This is because we intuitively believe it is wrong to do harm to others. However, it is not always clear, in research settings, when disadvantages outweigh advantages: in other words, a minor harm may sometimes be offset by a greater good. However, in line with the Nuremberg Code, this argument only has force when it is applied to a single individual. It is unethical to do all but the most trivial harm (say, taking a small blood sample) to a research subject for the benefit of others alone. But what if that injection is associated with a test for an illness for which there is currently no known cure? This might be considered an unacceptable level of harm if there were further harmful consequences for the person (e.g. psychological distress; risk of exclusion from medical or life insurance) if the test proved positive. Of course, if the illness is curable, or if there is some other clear benefit to the person, then the harm is possibly offset by such a benefit to a considerable degree. Indeed, it might even be thought of as unjust to withhold such a test from someone.

Justice is essentially the requirement that a thing or activity be fairly distributed amongst people. As a result, researchers are required to ensure that all individuals have an equal chance of being included from a study or benefiting from its results. For example, it is obviously unjust to exclude people from a study on the basis of race, colour, gender, age and so on. It is also unjust to exclude people, however, on the basis of other personal characteristics. One issue which affects researchers is the issue of linguistic preference or ability. It is typical to see researchers attempting to exclude from studies people whose first language is not English, or who have difficulties with writing and understanding written English. This means that these individuals do not benefit from the opportunity to participate in such studies, and is, therefore unfair or unjust towards them. It also has a further unjust consequence in that the study will then be carried out, for example, exclusively on people whose first language is English, and that results of the study will then be applied to those whose first language is *not*. Because they may differ from the English speakers in terms of other personal characteristics, this generalisation may be inappropriate and, therefore, unjust. Once again, there are potential grey areas here, because there are many languages for which validated measures have not yet been developed. It would be unwise to stop doing all research which involved such measures until they had been developed in all relevant languages, and would probably do, on balance, more harm than continuing to conduct such studies. At the same time, the research community has a responsibility to ensure that, wherever possible, adequate provision is made for non-English speakers and people who have difficulty with the written language, as well as continuing to develop scales which will be accessible by all.

These four principles inform the appropriate conduct of many aspects of research activity. Because they are so broad, their application is a matter of interpretation and judgement. It is also often difficult for researchers (who are not necessarily experts in ethics) to see precisely how they apply to their own studies. As a consequence, RECs seek to apply these principles on a case-by-case basis, usually in line with detailed criteria derived from these general notions.

Ethics and patient and public involvement in research

There are compelling reasons why we should wish to involve patients and the public in having a say in what research is conducted and how it is conducted. These reasons spring from all four of the principles outlined above.

If people wish to be involved in research, it is an offence to their autonomy if we do not allow them to do so as broadly as they might wish.

It is also offering them something of value, and so is an act of benefi-cence. More importantly, perhaps, to refuse to allow patients and the public a say is indefensible because to do so is a clear act of harm – we are treating them merely as objects in the research, preventing them from making a contribution they might wish to make, and decreasing the likelihood that the research will be relevant to them. This last of-fence may lead to further very practical and severe harms if it leads patients and the public to ignore results of beneficial research.

Finally, exclusion is unjust because it is unfair to exclude a particular group from participation on the basis of some irrelevant characteristic. In this case, the characteristic researchers have most often used to ex-clude patients and the public is that of lack of expertise in the subject matter. However, this is inappropriate in two ways: it is based on an assumption that technical expertise is necessary for making a contribu-tion to research (it isn't – such expertise is only necessary for specific methodological issues); it is based on too narrow a definition of exper-tise – for example, patients and the public have plentiful expertise in many areas, such as their experience of illness, even if we exclude the fact that many have become expert in the more traditional academic sense.

User involvement does, however, give rise to ethical issues in it-self, most often when patients are acting as members of the research team in a way which involves contact with patients. The argument has been advanced that this is problematic mainly because (a) patients who are researchers (often called *user-researchers)* might know other patients whom they then interact with as researchers, and that this would be an infringement of the privacy of this second 'researched' group and (b) user-researchers might be upset because of exposure to sensitive infor-mation during the course of their research role. The ethical offences in (a) and (b) are purported to be against autonomy and non-maleficence, respectively.

However, if taken as arguments against user involvement, both these arguments, in our view, lack any ethical force. This is because they are based on the view that *users* as researchers are in some relevant way different from any other researcher, and that this difference leads to dif-ferent conclusions about the ethical consequences for research subjects who come into contact with them and for the user-researchers them-selves. A moment's reflection reveals the problem with such a view. In (a), any researcher might come into contact with a subject whom they knew. In such an instance, we should expect them to behave appropri-ately, and the research protocol might even specify what they should do in such a case, in order to protect both researcher and subject. Nat-urally, we should expect any researcher to be advised or trained about what to do in such a case, and to respect confidentiality. There is no reason why we should not have similar expectations of, or offer sim-ilar advice and training, to a *user-researcher* as any other researcher.

Not to do so, incidentally, would be an offence against the principle of justice.

Equally, in (b) any researcher might become distressed by what they are researching and should be entitled to appropriate training, advice and support around such issues – user-researchers are not unique in this respect. Finally, this view neglects the fact that we are *all* patients or carers at some time in our lives. This in itself undermines the above argument that user-researchers are in some important way different from other researchers, unless we wish to suggest that no researcher who has had any health problem or cared for someone with such a problem can carry out health research.

Ethics committees and research governance

In essence, the broad principles of autonomy, beneficence and justice drive the work of RECs, which consider the ethical aspects of proposed research projects in healthcare. This work is co-ordinated under a central umbrella organisation: the National Research Ethics Service (NRES). NRES attempts to standardise the work of RECs, with the aim of ensuring that the level of ethical practice in research is similar across the UK[1]. The purpose of this standardisation is, ultimately, the protection of the public, specifically those individuals who become participants in research projects, but also, by ensuring that research is of a high standard, those people who eventually become users of the research, either as clinicians or patients. REC approval is also for the protection of the researchers themselves, because it provides a mechanism through which researchers can claim, in the event of any adverse event, that their research has been found to have reached certain minimum standards of ethical and methodological appropriateness.

All research work must receive REC approval before any data collection can begin, if that data collection involves any of the following: patients, relatives, staff, human tissue of any kind, access to patient records, use of National Health Service (NHS) premises. Additionally, approval may well be required if the researcher gains access to research participants by virtue of their role as a member of the NHS. For example, if you wished to interview mothers about the ways in which they gave medication to sick children, you could stand outside a school and stop them as they collected their children and offer them the chance to complete a questionnaire on such matters without seeking REC consent (although you would probably be unwise to do so unless you had some other robust system for ensuring the ethicality of the research). However, if you did exactly the same thing, but also told the parent that you were a health visitor working for such-and-such a primary care trust, you would definitely need REC consent, because you would be gaining access to the participants by virtue of your status as a health professional working in the NHS. The brief of RECs is to monitor and approve *all* NHS research activity, and it would be argued that your activity fell within this realm if you represented yourself as an NHS employee.

RECs are themselves now governed by a strict code of practice which is meant to ensure that their own conduct is ethical. The importance of this, from both an ethical and legal standpoint, has been the growth of a considerable bureaucracy around ethics committees in the UK and applications by researchers to them. This has resulted in occasional frustration by researchers with ethics committees, and a feeling that such committees were a barrier to the conduct of research. However, ethics committees take the view that the protection of the public is paramount. At the same time they recognise that harm would also be done if no research took place, and try extremely hard to balance these two issues in a way which is fair to both researchers and the public.

This bureaucracy has led to the development of a single national application form and procedure to be completed by all researchers who need REC approval, and this process is mediated via the internet. Although student research receives a slightly different from of scrutiny from RECs, students undergo the same application procedure as experienced researchers undertaking large funded research projects. The rationale for this is simple – although the work of students may not be far-reaching in its effects on the public, its potential for causing harm to individual participants is not necessarily less than the potential in a major research project. People requiring REC approval are advised to prepare the document in good time, and the approval process can take up to 60 days. If you are interested in finding out more about the role of RECs, particularly if you think will be undertaking a study which requires approval, full information can be found on the NRES website (see the end of this chapter for details).

A further step in the process of gaining approval for a study is the need to seek *Research Governance* approval. This is obtained from the research office of any NHS institution in which the research is to be carried out. Hospital Trusts each have their own research office, but Primary Care Trusts and smaller mental health Trusts often share research governance arrangements between several trusts. Strictly speaking, research offices do not consider ethical issues, but examine whether a study is feasible in their setting or has any potential financial impact on the host Trust. However, there are implicit ethical issues in many of the things to be considered in granting research governance approval. For example, if there is a financial impact, this may divert money away from patient care. Similarly, if the arrangements for research sponsorship are inadequate (research sponsors act as guarantors for the good ethical, financial and practical governance of research projects for which they are sponsors), there is potential for harm to participants. Whilst the general role of each research office in considering applications for research governance is similar, there is no centralised application system, and different Trusts have interpreted their responsibilities in ensuring the good governance of research activities in different ways, resulting in different documentation and different levels of scrutiny in different settings. Therefore, the seeking of research governance for a large, multicentre study can be extremely challenging, even for large teams of experienced researchers.

What can you do?

Given the above description of the complexities of REC and research governance approval, you might justifiably wonder how you could possibly have the time or resources to become involved in any research at all. There are a few things we would say in response to this. First, do not try and do it on your own. If you are intending to do a piece of your own research, you need supervision with this, and a competent supervisor will be familiar with REC and research governance issues.

Second, as a novice researcher, you should be starting small, and so issues about NHS ethics and research governance approval probably will not apply to you. If not, and you are a student, your university will almost certainly have its own ethics procedures. Although these differ widely in different universities, some form of procedure is essential, not just to protect subjects, but also to protect you as a researcher from possible risk of complaint or legal action if something goes wrong during the research. Most university procedures are considerably easier to negotiate than the NHS, which reflects the fact that the studies they are involved with are usually less risky and raise fewer ethical issues than those carried out with patients. One particular point you should note is that, at the time of writing this second edition, there is still no centralised agreed process for ethical scrutiny of studies which are carried out in non NHS hospital settings. You can seek advice from the setting where you propose to carry out the research, but should probably also make sure that your project has been seen by a university ethics committee. In social care settings, there is a single social care REC covering the country, but researchers are only required to apply to it if their research involves people who may lack capacity (although some funding bodies require applications to the social care REC for other groups of research participants). Otherwise, researchers are advised to apply to their university REC. If you are researching in a sensitive area (and, here again, as a novice researcher, you would be unwise to do so without the help of an experienced supervisor), it is worth seeking advice from an NHS REC, even when you are not required to do so. NHS RECs can offer advice and give an ethics opinion on any research, although the willingness to do so may vary from one local committee to another.

Finally, involvement in research goes far beyond the carrying out of pieces of research involving contact with patients, or even the collection of data from participants at all. There are many highly respected researchers who have confined their activities almost entirely to carrying out reviews of published source material. Moreover, activity in research, for most of us, is about critical understanding and dissemination and implementation. This is well within the scope of every HCP and is an extremely valuable contribution both to research itself and to patient care. The rest of this book will offer you an introduction to the skills needed to make a contribution in whatever way is most appropriate for you at the moment.

Review questions

What are the four principles, and why are they important? Is one more important than the rest?
When is approval from an NHS REC required?

Exercise

Have another look at the issues identified by the Nuremberg Code. Then, take the four principles of autonomy, beneficence, non-maleficence and justice and examine how the relate to each point of the code. Finally, consider how the four principles apply in the following situations:

You want to survey your own patients about their views of the care you have given.
One of your teachers or managers wants to interview you about your views of your course/job.

Endnote

1. Although healthcare is organised slightly differently in England and Wales, Scotland and Northern Ireland, the provision for healthcare research ethics scrutiny is essentially the same. Readers outside the UK will need to become aware of their national ethics provisions where these exist. However, the broad requirements are essentially similar, in that a review by an independent review body is always required.

References

Beauchamp, T. and Childress, J. (2001) *Principles of Biomedical Ethics*, 5th edn. Oxford: Oxford University Press.

Gillon, R. (2003) 'Ethics needs principles – four can encompass the rest – and respect for autonomy should be "first among equals"'. *Journal of Medical Ethics*, 29, 307–312.

Further reading

Milgram, S. (1963). Behavioral study of obedience. *Journal of Abnormal and Social Psychology*, 67, 371–378.

Nuremberg doctors' trial (1996) *British Medical Journal*, 313, 1448. Also available online at http://bmj.bmjjournals.com/cgi/content/full/313/7070/1448

Rosenhan, D. (1975) On being sane in insane places. *Science*, 179, 250–258.

Websites

http://www2.carleton.ca/secretariat/policies/the-ethical-conduct-of-research/

http://www.dh.gov.uk/en/Researchanddevelopment/A-Z/Researchgovernance/index.htm

http://www.mrc.ac.uk/Newspublications/Publications/Ethicsandguidance/index.htm

http://www.nres.npsa.nhs.uk/

Basic Concepts: Sampling, Reliability and Validity

6

Key points

- Sampling is an everyday activity, not peculiar to research.
- A population is a total group from which a sample is drawn.
- Some populations are themselves samples from larger populations.
- Representativeness is the key to sampling, but is defined differently by quantitative and qualitative researchers.
- Samples may be random or non-random.
- Sampling technique is guided by the aim of the research.
- Validity is the extent to which a study examines the entity it says it does.
- Reliability is that it does so in a systematised, repeatable way.
- Quantitative and qualitative researchers place different emphasis on different aspects of validity and reliability.

Sampling in research

This chapter introduces the ideas of reliability and validity in the context of what it means to sample from a wider population. In Chapter 3, we noted that different methodological approaches often have

Research for Evidence-Based Practice in Healthcare, Second edition, by Robert Newell and Philip Burnard
© 2011 Robert Newell and Philip Burnard

different research aims associated with them. In the same way, the different approaches and aims are generally associated with different ways of sampling. However, perhaps the most basic distinction in sampling in research is the one between sampling in quantitative and qualitative research. The specifics of different sampling techniques used in qualitative and quantitative approaches are examined in detail in Chapters 7 and 13.

In this chapter, basic notions of the *rationale behind* sampling are explored. We start from a quantitative perspective because this is the one most commonly encountered in medical and healthcare research studies. Even when a qualitative study is reported in the literature, the sampling technique may still be one initially derived from quantitative approaches. We also believe that the notion of sampling is not peculiar to research, but is part of our everyday lives, and many of our everyday concepts of sampling are most easily understood from a quantitative perspective. At the same time, we do not ignore qualitative perspectives on sampling, and you will see these are mentioned throughout this chapter.

Samples and populations

Most of us are familiar with the national census. Infrequently, the whole population of the UK is presented with a series of forms to fill in, asking for information about their characteristics. The sheer size of this undertaking is so vast that it only takes place once every 10 years. In between times, things change, and government organisations continue to need information which reflects those changes. In the absence of resources to repeat the *whole population* census or survey, smaller surveys are conducted on a limited *sample* of the population. Similarly, in most research studies, it would be very difficult to survey, say, every person who had undergone a hernia operation and ask them about their satisfaction with care. In this situation, health researchers follow the same approach as these government surveys, and sample a certain number of patients.

In both these examples, we make the assumption that the sample is similar to the population from which it is drawn. In the first case, this is the population of all people in the UK; in the second, it is the population of all people who have had hernia operations. This is also the commonsense way in which we typically talk about samples and populations. Nor is this simply a consequence of our having been brought up with scientific jargon thrust on us from school onwards, via teachers and the media. For example, the New Testament story of Jesus begins with a survey. Mary and Joseph travel to Bethlehem essentially to be counted for tax purposes.

Sampling as an everyday pursuit

In our own experience, we think implicitly in terms of populations and samples. Imagine you wanted to get wedding photos taken, or special 50th Wedding Anniversary photos for your parents. The consequences of making the wrong choice of photographer are potentially expensive, both financially and emotionally. Before employing a photographer, you will probably ask to see a sample of her work. You might actually go to several photographers in the neighbourhood getting sample photographs from each, before finally deciding. When you do both these things, you are actually making a number of sophisticated sampling decisions which are precisely similar to the decisions faced by researchers.

Consider the following issues. When you ask to see samples of a photographer's work, you expect that these will be reflective of all the photographs (the population of photographs) she has taken. Of course, you accept that she will have chosen her best work to show you, but that probably matters less to you than seeing the *kind* of photos she takes. If she specialises in highly formal posed shots, her sample will reflect that, and that information is useful to you in making your decision because you assume it is reflective of her work as a whole. As we will see later, you have accepted that the sample will not be *random* but will be selected by the photographer in a *non-random* way. This, however, does not concern you because the issue you are concerned with (style of photos) is not dependent on randomness to be an adequate sample of the photographer's work (unless she takes photographs in different styles and has chosen to show you only one such style). Many sampling decisions in research are variants of these two issues: What characteristics of the population do I wish to capture in the sample? What approach to sampling will best capture these?

One aspect of decision making about sampling we have not covered so far is the notion of what one's aim is in capturing particular characteristics of the population in the sample. Yet, in the photograph example, this point emerges readily. Your aim, of course, is to get the best possible set of pictures for your wedding or your parents, *given the circumstances*. These circumstances give rise to a whole series of further sampling decisions. To give just two examples of circumstances that affect our sampling decisions, what you really are aiming for in this example is to get the best possible set of photographs *within a reasonable time, at a price you can afford*. Because of the need to meet the *reasonable time* aim, you need only sample from photographers you know do not have a long waiting list. Similarly, to meet this aim, it will only be practical to sample a certain number of photographers (perhaps only those in your nearest large town or nearest city). Finally, to satisfy the *at a price you can afford* aim, there is no point in sampling from photographers whose work you know you cannot afford.

If your aim is different, your approach to sampling will be different. If you want to know what kind of range of wedding photographs exists (say, because you have not seen many and want to see what different sorts look like), you will no longer be concerned with the *at a price I can afford* goal. You just want to know about style, not about price, because you are not buying yet, although price may affect your decision later. The *within a reasonable time* goal does not concern you much either (except if you spend so long looking at wedding photos that you run out of time before the wedding!). In this situation, you are much more likely to want a broad ranging sample. First, you probably want a random selection of each photographer's work, rather than ones that photographer thinks are suitable for you. Second, you will want to see the work of a great many photographers, not just local ones. You may even go so far as to take a random sample of all UK photographers, if time and money are no object. This is because you are aware that the broader the sample, the better, in giving you responses which are broad ranging.

Finally, your first concern might be to engage a photographer who is sympathetic to the needs of bride and groom on their wedding day, or your parents on the day of their 50th Wedding Anniversary. In this situation, your sample may be very much smaller than in the second example we gave above, because the kind of information you want from them may be very detailed, which in turn will affect the amount of time it takes you to gather it from them. In this case, you may decide on personal visits from a small range of local photographers, during which you discuss the event, their approach to it, and also get an idea of their personality. Here, you have accepted that the sample is likely to be quite unreflective of the whole population of photographers, or even photographers in your town for hire at a good price, because you believe this disadvantage in your approach to sampling is offset by the advantage to you in gaining the very detailed information you need from a few respondents.

In each of these situations, our ideas about sampling are different because of the different aims we have. We also adjust our ideas of what constitutes the population. In the first example, we have defined the population as wedding photographers who can do the job in a reasonable time, in the second as all photographers, and in the third as local photographers. Naturally, as you will have gathered from the above, all these supposed populations are actually themselves samples. For example, wedding photographers are themselves a subsample of the population of all professional photographers, who are again a subsample of the population of all photographers. This is where confusion sometimes arises, but is best settled by considering a sample to be a smaller element examined from some larger entity. The population is that larger entity, but may itself be a smaller element of some still larger entity. Ultimately, all photographers are simply a sample of a broader population of all human beings. We define the population according to our needs, and sample from it in the same way.

Turning to healthcare, the sampling decisions we took above are also evident in much health research. We may, for example, survey hernia patients in our own hospital, even if we know that that hospital's approach to hernia repair and its care is very different from many other hospitals' care. If our aim is simply to monitor and improve care in our own hospital, that does not matter. If we wish to make some broader claim (say, about the best way to organise care for hernia patients *in general*) we will accept the inconvenience of having take a broader sample, perhaps choosing other hospitals to sample from on a random basis, and employing some systematic form of sampling within each institution. On the other hand, if we are at a stage where we want detailed accounts of the patient's experience of the patient journey in repair of hernias, including what their impressions were of what happened to them, their feelings at the time, their attitudes to others around them, the atmosphere on the ward while they were being treated, and so on, our decision will be similar to the one described in our description of the search for a sympathetic photographer. We will choose a very few people, gain a great deal of information from them and accept that this information may be particular to them rather than reflective of the personal experiences of hernia repair patients as a whole. Naturally, we would probably also want to argue that the insights we had gained from them would be useful in considering the possible experiences of others, but the rationale we gave for making such an assertion would not be on grounds of the way in which the individuals in the sample might reflect individuals in the population at large.

Samples and representativeness

On several occasions, we have described samples as being more or less reflective of the populations from which they are drawn. This is the concept of representativeness and is a basic notion in sampling. Roadside breathalyser tests measure alcohol levels in the human body. If it were the case that the sample of such levels did not represent the levels present in a person's body as a whole, there would be little chance of gaining a conviction for drink driving, and we should agree that this would be fair enough, because the sample would not be telling us about the actual *population of* alcohol levels in that person's body at the time. Indeed, there have been a number of recent celebrated court cases in which contamination of human tissue samples has led to the acquittal of the accused. These cases are essentially examples of situations where there could be no confidence that the samples were truly representative of the *population of* that person's tissue.

Once again, if we extend this idea to healthcare practice, we can see that it would be futile to base interventions on samples that were not representative of the whole. If a blood sample is not representative of the patient's blood as a whole, it does not tell us much about the population (all that patient's blood) or, by extension, about their health status. The same is true of psychological measures. If we measure a person's level of depression using an accepted scale, we do so because we believe that the scale gives us a meaningful sample of their mood, and base our interventions on its results. This is because we are confident that the scale results are representative of the patient's mood as a whole (the population of their mood levels, if you like).

In qualitative research, many researchers have wanted to deny the importance of representativeness. This argument is often misunderstood, however. Qualitative researchers are certainly concerned with representativeness, even when they wish only to describe the experiences of their participant group, rather than drawing inferences from that group to a wider population. This is because they will want us to have confidence that the responses they have gained from their participants are, in fact, representative of what their respondents think (in other words, that they are a representative sample of those people's thoughts). The central difference between approaches to representativeness in quantitative and qualitative research is that the two traditions emphasise different issues in defining representativeness.

In quantitative research, our confidence in representativeness comes overwhelmingly from sampling technique. Have we sampled in such a way that we can be sure that this individual, or this sample of blood, is truly representative of the population from which we claim to have drawn it? In qualitative research, we are more likely to be concerned with theoretical issues. Do the responses genuinely reflect some characteristic of the whole? In our photography examples, both quantitative and qualitative concerns are reflected in the first example. We want a representative sample of photographers (albeit within certain constraints). However, we are not concerned that the examples of their work may be non-random because, whatever the sample they choose, we know it represents a theoretically important aspect of their work – their style. In the second example, quantitative notions prevail. Representativeness of the sample is the key element, and all our efforts will be geared to ensuring this (see Chapter 14). Finally, in the third example, our approach is very much at the qualitative end of the spectrum in sampling terms. There is no representativeness of the sample from the quantitative perspective, but it is fit for the researcher's purpose, because it allows the in-depth exploration necessary to bring to the surface issues of concern to the researcher. Moreover, the researcher does not need to worry that the responses of the participants will not be representative of the broader range of their thoughts, feelings and attitudes. Provided the information is sensitively gathered, the responses will, by definition, bring to the surface aspects of the photographer's personality and so on, and this is the information required by you in this context.

Validity and reliability

Both qualitative and quantitative research are concerned with the principles of validity and reliability, although, as we shall see in Chapters 12, 13 and 14, the two research approaches have slightly different criteria for determining these and sometimes different terminology to reflect the underlying constructs. Nevertheless, qualitative and quantitative researchers are generally united in the view that the entity being examined (rather than something else) should emerge from the results of a study (validity) and that it should do so in a systematised way (reliability).

Validity refers to several ways in which we can be confident that the thing under investigation is truly emerging. Thus, we speak of a measure as having validity if it genuinely measures the thing it claims to measure. A structured interview which claimed to measure quality of life, but actually measured depression levels would be an invalid measure of quality of life, because low mood is only one part of this. Any conclusions we drew about quality of life based on such a measure would likewise be invalid. We also describe research studies as having validity. Typically, this terminology has been borrowed and extended from experimental research and is discussed in more detail in Chapters 13 and 14.

Reliability is the extent to which an entity is measured in a consistent way. To be reliable, a measure needs to be repeatable (giving similar responses in the same conditions) and reproducible (giving similar responses in different conditions).

Validity, reliability and sampling

Internal validity refers to our confidence that changes in a patient's status are caused by the treatment they are given, rather than some extraneous event (upbringing, personality, genetic inheritance) and is greatly increased by the use of random sampling (see Chapters 14, 15 and 18). In this situation, adequate sampling increases confidence that we are truly measuring the relationship between treatment and changes in patient status – the thing we claim to be measuring.

The notion of external validity is related to generalisability and refers to how confident we can be that results found in our sample reflect attributes of the population. As we suggested in the photography example, we are not always concerned with this, and the more tightly we define the sample and population, the more we decrease external validity. For example, one enduring criticism of randomised controlled trials (see Chapter 17) is that, although participants may have been randomly sampled from the population concerned (thus increasing internal validity), the population (e.g. males between 18 and 65 with no other illnesses attending South of England teaching hospitals and willing to participate) is itself so untypical that generalisability to the greater population of hernia repair patients is low. In this situation, selective sampling decreases external validity. Validity is low if we claim the study is genuinely measuring the responses of all hernia repair patients.

Reliability in sampling extends the idea of reliability of measurement by asking if the sampling strategy and techniques collect from the population in a replicable way. For a sampling strategy to be reliable, it should garner the same results from a population every time we sample, provided the attribute being examined remains unchanged. In most situations, a random sampling approach is an important beginning in ensuring such reliability of results, but other issues such as interviewer technique and instrument reliability also impact heavily on reliability of data collection. Although they seem unrelated to sampling itself, actually there are obvious relationships between sampling approach and data collection approach and technique. For example, there would be little point in taking a random sample of cancer patients if we wanted to undertake, say, a dozen in-depth interviews with them about their experiences of delays in diagnosis and treatment. A random sample with such a small number would never give us sufficient participants who had experienced delays *and* could talk in depth about them *and* had a broad range of experiences, but the use of in-depth interviews is arguably the most reliable way of getting such information.

Horses for courses

This final point gives us, once again, the key feature of approaches to sampling. There are no right and wrong ways to sampling, only more and less appropriate ones under any given set of circumstances. Appropriate sampling should reflect the aims of the research study, as well as the practical constraints under which the study takes place. Our decisions about sampling take place within these two contexts.

Review questions

What is the difference between a population and a sample?
When and why does representativeness matter?
What do we mean by validity and reliability in sampling?

> **Exercise**
>
> Sampling is an everyday pursuit. Consider three occasions in your own non-work life when you have undertaken informal sampling. What was your purpose? Was the sampling random or non-random? How did this affect its usefulness?

Further reading

Burns, N. and Grove, S.K. (2004) *The Practice of Nursing Research*, 5th edn. Philadelphia: Saunders.

Website

http://www.depauloresearch.com/sampsize.htm

SECTION 2
Qualitative Approaches

Issues in Qualitative Data Collection

Key points

- Data collection choices are made in response to research aims.
- Sampling in qualitative research aims at illumination rather than representativeness.
- Interviews may be structured, semi-structured or unstructured.
- Interviews are normally transcribed verbatim.
- Sometimes qualitative data can be gleaned from questionnaires.
- Observational studies benefit from painstaking field notes.
- Published work can be subjected to similar data analysis to other research methods.

Introduction

The first question when deciding on a data collection method is this: 'What sort of data will help me to answer my research question or achieve my research aims?' The second question is then: 'What is the

Research for Evidence-Based Practice in Healthcare, Second edition, by Robert Newell and Philip Burnard
© 2011 Robert Newell and Philip Burnard

most appropriate method for collecting those data?' This chapter considers issues related to collecting qualitative data.

As we noted in Chapter 3, it is always the research question that determines the method. There is a danger, sometimes, in researchers limiting themselves, when writing their research questions, by having half an eye on the methods they *want* to use. If we want to be honest and clear in doing research, we need, first, to formulate our question very clearly and only then decide on method. For the purposes of the rest of the chapter, it is supposed that the researcher has done this and has decided that qualitative data are needed. As we have seen in other chapters, the form of these data is usually textual. Qualitative research is normally about the generation and analysis of words. Those words can take at least three forms: words uttered in interviews, words written down by the researcher following or during observation or words that are already published. Following an examination of sampling issues which might affect the collection of these forms of words, we will look at how each different form of words might be gathered.

Sampling for qualitative research

It should be noted that whilst an aim in quantitative research is usually to generalise from the findings (and this is often possible because of the nature of the sampling used), the aim of qualitative research is *not* to generalise (because the nature of the sampling and the methods of data collection and analysis do not allow it). This is an important point that must always be borne in mind when reporting qualitative findings. Nevertheless, the findings from qualitative samples may be illustrative of particular experiences and points of view. Indeed, the kind of sampling and data collection strategies employed by qualitative researchers often allow very detailed and deep descriptions of personal accounts.

In Chapter 2, we touched on three popular forms of sampling for qualitative research: convenience sampling, purposive sampling and snowball sampling. We noted that convenience sampling involved sampling from people who happened to be available to participate, whilst purposive sampling involved selecting people on the basis of their being likely to have things to say relevant to the research aim, and snowball sampling was a particular variant of purposive sampling involving having respondents themselves recommend potential additional respondents. None of these approaches to sampling attempt to be representative. However, as we saw in Chapter 6, this is not necessarily a drawback.

Popular sampling strategies in qualitative research

Convenience sampling – participants are readily available, but members of the sample may not be best respondents.

Purposive sampling – deliberately selects those who are likely to have most to say.

Snowball sampling – allows selection of likely candidates from difficult to reach groups.

Whilst convenience sampling perhaps has least to recommend it, it still has distinct advantages, not least of which is that participants are readily available. This may be a compelling advantage for hard pressed students with limited resources. The great disadvantage, however, is that members of a convenience sample may have little to say of use in the illumination of the research question. For example, an examination of the experiences of social workers of working with people with drug problems might run into this issue of relevance if our convenience sample contained only social workers who had limited experience of caring for such clients. In a quantitative study, we might be able to make use of their limited responses, but for qualitative research, it is unlikely we would get the kind of detailed personal accounts which are at the heart of the qualitative approach to research. On the other hand, almost any convenience sample of social workers could give us such detailed accounts of their experiences of having been students. In such a situation, the weaknesses of a convenience sample would be trivial compared with the great advantage of availability.

Where the phenomena we want to study are fairly common, then, a convenience approach has a lot to recommend it. However, the more unusual the phenomenon, the more likely it is that we will want to turn to purposive sampling as a way of recruiting people with relevant information. In purposive sampling, the researcher sets out a specific set of criteria according to which participants will be selected, and then recruits as many participants as are required who meet these criteria. Often, purposive sampling is highly selective, resulting in a unique group of individuals, and it may be that all available participants are recruited. Patton (1990) has suggested a considerable number of differing purposes for purposive sampling, dependent on the differing possible aims of the researcher. For example, during a project, the search for deviant cases (who point to unusual aspect of the issue under study), typical cases (who show typical examples of the issue), theory-based cases (who demonstrate characteristics in line with a particular theory and so allow us to expand upon that theory) are all types of purposive searching for participants. About 20 other types of purposive sampling are identified in Patton's book.

Sometimes, it is difficult to find a way into a particular cultural group (drug users, abused women, criminals). Once again, a form of purposive sampling is a useful tool for the qualitative researcher. In this case, snowball sampling is the approach of choice. It relies on the idea that people in particular communities are best placed to direct the researcher to potential sources of further information. The more closed or covert the community, the more likely it is that the researcher will need to make use of the snowball approach, but at the same time, the more difficult this will become, because the research will need to work hard to gain the trust of initial respondents, so that they will feel comfortable in commending the researcher to other potential participants. However, once that trust is gained, the snowball approach is a powerful way of gaining information from hard-to-reach participant groups. There is, however, an ethical dilemma in some instances of the use of snowballing with hard-to-reach groups. This is the possibility that harm may come to a respondent as a result of putting the researcher in contact with other potential participants. The case of criminal behaviour is an obvious example. A potential respondent may be less than happy about having their status as one who engages in illegal activities revealed to a third party in the form of a researcher whose pedigree and motivations are unknown to them.

It is impossible to give an immediate illustration of a typical size of a sample in quantitative research. Typical sizes of samples in qualitative research range from a single case to about 30 respondents. The literature offers little conclusive evidence of the importance of particular sample sizes in qualitative research. One method that is sometimes used to limit samples in qualitative studies is to continue to interview respondents, or collect other forms of data, until the same information starts being repeated over and over again with no new information emerging. This is sometimes referred to as 'saturation'. Interviews or other forms of data collection can stop at this point and thus the sample size is limited by the nature of the forthcoming data. Naturally, it takes considerable skill and experience to reach a reasonable decision as to when no new information is likely to emerge.

Sample size in qualitative research

There is little definitive guidance on sample size in qualitative research.

For in-depth examination of data, it is rare for more than 30 respondents to be used.

Saturation can help decide sample size but is itself hard to recognise.

Could qualitative researchers use randomised samples?

The standard view on qualitative sampling is that it is not necessary to use a random sample. Qualitative research, so the argument goes, reflects personal, subjective reporting of personal, subjective data. However, it is possible to question this point of view.

One of the reasons that qualitative findings cannot be generalised is because of the sampling methods used. In the past, qualitative researchers had to do most things by hand. They wrote down interviews and then analysed them – also by hand. Today, there are many technologies that help make the data collection and data analysis processes easier. Clearly, interviews can be recorded. They can also be analysed with the aid of computer programs. Such programs do not *do* the analysis but are a potent aid to the process. Such programs can work with computer-based transcripts of interviews or even with the direct voice-recordings of those interviews.

All this raises the tentative question as to whether or not large-scale qualitative studies, involving randomised samples might be conducted, from which the findings could be generalised. Some view this idea as heresay or as a plain misunderstanding of the nature of qualitative research. Like most things, however, it is worth thinking about.

Interviews and focus groups

In qualitative research, three types of interviews can be noted: structure, semi-structured and unstructured. Along that continuum comes an increasing difficulty in later analysis. Structured interviews are probably the easiest to analyse (or, perhaps, to 'organise'). Semi-structured interviews are rather more difficult and unstructured interviews can become so wayward that they can be very difficult – if not impossible – to analyse. However, in terms of value and usefulness, the gradient seems, sometimes, to be reversed: unstructured interviews can sometimes lead us closer to other people's meaning systems, whilst structured ones can be very arid affairs. Another method of data collection is the 'group interview' or focus group.

The structured interview

This form of interview can be likened to a sort of 'verbal questionnaire'. The research prepares a list of questions which the interviewee then answers. No leeway is given for alternative questions or for any further ones. It is usually important that the interview schedules that are prepared for these interviews contain, almost exclusively, *open* questions (as opposed to *closed* questions). A closed question is one that elicits only a one word answer – and very often, the answer is either 'yes' or 'no'. On the other hand, an open question is broader and asks the interviewee to express a view or an opinion. If *only* closed questions are to be asked, then the research needs to consider if it would not be more economical of time and energy to use a questionnaire rather than an interview. Moreover, the data gathered from such closed questions is hardly in keeping with the spirit of qualitative research.

The big advantage of the structured interview is in the marshalling of the data, afterwards. The responses to each question, from each interviewee, can be brought together and reported. A particularly straightforward way of doing this is, for reporting purposes, to turn the question used in the interview, into a statement. Thus, if the question was 'What are your views about the value of reflective practice in the clinical setting?', it is turned, in the report, into the heading: 'Student's views of the value of reflective practice in the clinical setting'.

The big disadvantage is that the structured interview does not allow the interview room to encourage the interviewee to expand on what they have to say. The researcher is limited to only asking the questions as they appear on the interview schedule. The structured interview is useful, in a large-scale project, if a number of interviewers (apart from the researcher) are to be trained to collect data. The structure ensures that data of a similar sort will routinely be collected from each respondent – despite the fact that different interviewers are being used. This approach is often used for large-scale surveys and opinion polls.

Semi-structured interviews

This is a variant on the above approach. The researcher who uses the semi-structured approach has a series of questions that they wish to ask. Or, they may have a series of topics in mind, around which they will frame questions. However, the researcher is also prepared to ask subsequent questions and to use prompts to encourage the interviewee to say more. A decision may also be made not necessarily to ask the questions in a particular order but to change the order according to the respondents' responses. This approach encourages the interview to flow more freely: one topic often leads, seamlessly, into another until the interviewer has covered all her questions. The general aim is to cover *similar* territory, in each interview, but not to control the interview to the degree that each respondent is asked exactly the same questions in exactly the same order.

The researcher needs to practice this method before she uses it and some counselling skills training can sometimes be helpful in encouraging the researcher to use prompts and other devices to help the respondent to keep talking. However, there is an important difference in the *aim* of counselling and data collection. While counselling is mostly about helping a person to talk about their problems and helping them sort out those problems, the aim of the research interview is to collect data. The research interview is never, in any sense, a form of counselling or therapy. Indeed, if the issues under discussion are sensitive, the researcher should have contingency plans to cover what happens if the respondent becomes upset. It is not normally ethically justifiable to continue to gather data when a person is upset, nor may it be justifiable to use the data so collected.

Excerpt from a semi-structured interview

Researcher: 'What do you think are the advantages of reflective practice?'

Respondent: 'Well, I don't know really. I suppose you could say that it makes you think more carefully about your work. Like what you do when you are in the ward ... you have to be careful though, really ...'

Researcher: 'You have to be careful?'

Respondent: 'Yes. I remember our lecturer going on about 'reflection in action'. Well, if we did that, we would have all sorts of problems! I mean you can't just always reflect on things as you do them. It would be really difficult and cause loads of problems'.

Researcher: 'Can you give me an example of some of the problems?'

Respondent: 'Well, imagine you are working in theatre and the doctors are doing this big operation and you are like handling some of the instruments and counting and so on. Imagine if you do reflection in action while you are doing that! You need to be able to concentrate!'

Researcher: 'Concentrate ...'

Respondent: 'You need to be like focussed on what you are doing. Not thinking about it but just doing it. You have been trained and you know why you are doing it. I can't see the point in just reflecting more on it – especially in theatre or something.'

Here, the researcher has used a single, scheduled question and then a variety of prompts and reflections to encourage the respondent to say more and to elaborate on a theme. The researcher does not offer his or her own views but encourages the respondent to answer the original question in more depth. Clearly, it is important to appreciate when to do this and when not to. There is always a danger of 'bucketing an empty well' and searching for elaboration when no elaboration is in the head of the respondent. To do this runs the risk of the respondent merely saying things for the sake of saying them or even making up responses to satisfy the researcher. The researcher, then, should prompt without being intrusive.

Notice, in the above example, the respondent uses vernacular speech – including many examples of the 'filler' word 'like'. There is a debate amongst researchers as to whether or not researchers should report data from respondents keeping this style of speech intact, or whether the research should attempt to 'tidy up' the language of the respondent. Probably, most involved in the debate favour the former view: that the utterances should be reported, as they are and that no attempt should be made to exclude colloquialisms pauses, repetitions and so on.

Unstructured interviews

These normally start from the same point but can end in any number of places. The researcher usually starts the interview with a broad, open question (e.g., 'what are your thoughts about student grants?'). From the response to this, the researcher encourages the interviewee to say more and does not attempt to 'lead' the interview but allows it to follow the direction dictated by the respondent's utterances. One of the immediate dangers, of course, is that the interview can veer very much off course and away from the direct focus of the research study. In this way, many unstructured interviews slowly become more structured as the researcher feels compelled to bring the conversation back to firmer ground.

Again, techniques borrowed from counselling can be useful here. The researcher may use reflection or echoing and repeat the last few words of a respondent's utterance to encourage him or her to continue speaking, without breaking a chain of thought. The researcher may summarise what the respondent has said, so far, in order (a) to check the degree to which he or she (the researcher) has understood and (b) to help the respondent move on. These techniques, along with the use of further open questions, can be accompanied by all the behavioural techniques that show that the researcher is listening and that encourage the respondent to talk. These include the use of minimal prompts ('mm' and 'ok'), nods of the head and also the maintenance of reasonably sustained eye contact. However, it should be noted that there are huge cultural variations in what is considered appropriate eye contact, and these, too, should be noted and respected.

In the end, it is probable that most qualitative researchers, using the interview method of data collection, also use the semi-structured variant. As we have noted, structured interviews are very limiting and unstructured ones can become unwieldy and produce such diverse data that comparison and contrast between transcriptions can become difficult or impossible.

Other issues concerning interviews

The general advice given to those who interview in research is that interviews should be tape recorded. There are, however, at least two possibilities and the present author has used both effectively. One is to make hand-written notes during the interview or to have a colleague act as rapporteur. This is not as difficult as it sounds. In a recent study, in Thailand, the author found that tape recording of interviews was not practical. Thai people (in comparison to European people) talk quietly, accents were quite marked, and these issues, plus the noise from air conditioning all combined to make recordings unintelligible. After the first interview, the author simply asked questions and managed to copy, word-for-word, most of what was said. As direct eye-contact, in Thailand, is not very common, the activity of the researcher's writing also seemed to help, rather than hinder, the interview process. Sometimes, too, a co-researcher sat in on interviews and took notes.

A second alternative is to use a laptop computer to directly keyin answers to questions. This means, of course, that the researcher needs to be able to type quickly and, preferably, to touch-type. If the researcher *does* type quickly, it is quite possible to keep up with the utterances of the interviewee. We have used this method to transcribe telephone interviews as they were being conducted. We are less certain about the appropriateness of them in the face-to-face interview setting.

Focus groups

Focus group research has a considerable history in market research and, more recently, in politics. It was designed primarily to judge people's reactions to stimulus materials such as products and packaging, although that purpose was soon extended to include reactions to broader concepts or ideas. In classic focus group procedures, participants in groups which typically range between 6 and 12 people are shown some stimulus object and/or introduced to an idea by the use of 'trigger questions' to orientate them to issues to be examined. They then discuss these ideas with the assistance of a 'moderator' (basically a researcher with group leading experience) who directs the group interaction through questioning, reflection and summarising. As in individual interviews, the interactions are often audio-recorded, but, unlike in interviews, in focus groups there is often a second researcher who takes charge of the technical aspects of recording.

This method can be particularly useful in healthcare where we want to examine people's reactions to a piece of equipment, information materials, proposed or actual redesign of services and so on. Focus groups are frequently conducted by people working in healthcare who want to involve patients and carers in the design of services, or to seek their opinions on a broad range of issues relevant to healthcare provision. Increasingly, focus groups have come to be used more broadly still in healthcare research. Thus, they are often used not just to examine participants' reactions to some particular form of stimulus or issue, but also to ask them about their experiences in general.

It is regarded as a strength, rather than a weakness, of focus groups that group members influence each other during the course of the group. Thus, it is not necessarily a bad thing in focus group research if one group member is particularly dominant, or if another is especially passive. This part of what is observed and analysed in focus group research is the pattern of interaction between participants (the second researcher present may, in addition to handling technical aspects, observe these interactions during the group), and these interactions are taken into account in the analysis of data collected in the group. Naturally, the dominance over the group of a particular individual should not reach the extreme position where only that individual's views are heard, and it is part of the skill of the moderator to ensure that there is reasonable representation of all group members, both in the group itself and in the subsequent analysis. By the same token, focus group researchers recognise that vociferous, dominant members may have something important to say about the target issue. However, particularly in the case of focus groups which examine people's experiences, there is an equal and opposite position which suggests that, as each contributor's experiences are equally important, each should get an equal chance to express themselves.

This practical difficulty, in our view, is one potential limitation for the type of focus group which examines individual experiences, because the analysis of group interactions is difficult, and the impact of that interaction on individual members especially so. It is, therefore, potentially hard to unravel how far the reported experiences of one individual in a group are influenced by their co-members. For this reason, we prefer to distinguish between the focus group (which embodies the components of reaction to stimulus materials and analysis of interaction) from the group interview (which typically does not). As its name suggests, the group interview is basically a number of interviews asking about individual views, but conducted in a group setting, with relatively little examination of interactions. Here, the issue of the potential for bias as a result of dominant group members is clearly more problematic, because we claim to be primarily examining individual responses, not group responses. Much of the supposed focus group research we have seen, both at the proposal stage and in publication, actually looks much more like group interviewing, and is presented with little or no comment on interactions, either from the viewpoint of potential bias or as a source of enrichment of the emerging data.

More serious still is the suggestion that focus group research is an economical use of time, allowing the collection of large amounts of data in a short time. Once again, we have seen this asserted in both proposals for funding or ethics approval and in research reports. Yet a few seconds' contemplation will show this assertion to be false. If you do an hour of interviewing, you get an hour of data, whether you interview one individual during an hour or 100 during an hour. In fact, it is likely that you actually get less individual information in a group interview, because each participant gets less time to develop any ideas. It is for this reason that we suggest that focus group research should be confined to situations where there is either some clear stimulus material to be responded to (for instance, acceptability of a new questionnaire), or where examination of interactions is intended by the researchers.

Transcription

It is usually necessary to transcribe interviews or focus groups from tape recordings (or to type up notes). When this is done, it is best if a large margin can be allowed, on the right-hand edge of the text. This can be used, later, for notes during the process of content analysing the data (something that is discussed in another chapter). Thus, the text will look as follows:

Researcher: 'What do you think are the advantages of reflective practice?'

Respondent: 'Well, I don't know really. I suppose you could say that it makes you think more carefully about your work. Like what you do when you are in the ward ... you have to be careful though, really ...'

Researcher: 'You have to be careful?'

Respondent: 'Yes. I remember our lecturer going on about "reflection in action". Well, if we did that, we would have all sorts of problems! I mean you can't just always reflect on things as you do them. It would be really difficult and cause loads of problems'.

Researcher: 'Can you give me an example of some of the problems?'

Respondent: 'Well, imagine you are working in theatre and the doctors are doing this big operation and you are like handling some of the instruments and counting and so on. Imagine if you do reflection in action while you are doing that! You need to be able to concentrate!'

Researcher: 'Concentrate ...'

It is a matter of debate whether or not the researcher should always transcribe his or her own interviews. One view is that in transcribing the material, the researcher is able to get 'closer' to the data, through re-reading it. Another view is that transcription is a time-consuming (and often very boring) activity that can, where possible, be 'sub-contracted'. Finance also enters into this debate: clearly, not everyone will have the resources to pay another person to do data transcriptions. Also, all transcriptions that are typed by someone other than the researcher need very careful checking. There is, of course, a considerable difference between the 'heard' word and the written word. There is considerable room for error in the process of converting the spoken word into the written.

Another debate lies in whether or not *all* interviews should be transcribed (or, indeed, if *any* need to be). While most researchers seem to favour the transcription of all interviews, some feel that it is not necessary, always, to transcribe those undertaken towards the end of the data collection cycle. The argument is that in these later interviews much of what is said is likely to be a repetition of points made in earlier ones. Yet others feel that the bringing together of similar forms of data, in forms of content analysis, can be done by working directly with tape recordings. We have always made transcriptions of all interviews in qualitative studies and never found it possible to work directly from recordings. Accordingly, we do not recommend attempting to analyse untranscribed recordings to novice researchers.

Problems with the interview method

The interview method remains, perhaps, the most commonly used method of collecting qualitative research data. It is worth noting some of the problems associated with it. First, interviewer and respondent are interacting with each other. Each is, as it were, sizing each other up. Each is trying to work out what the other person is like. In this process, the respondent – in particular – is trying to work out, at some level, what the researcher wants to hear. He or she may not even be aware of doing this, but it is a feature of most interactions between two people. This can skew what the respondent says to this particular researcher at this particular time. If another person was conducting the interview, a different set of responses might be obtained. However, when findings from interviews are reported, little or no mention is made of what might be called the 'dynamics of the interview'. Findings are reported as if they, necessarily, represented the straightforward views of the person being interviewed. They are, though, a *particular* set of views that have arisen out of this particular interview.

Second, we are all subject to moods, changes of views and opinions. What we say today may not be what we would have said last week and may not be what we would want to say next month. In this respect, interviews are rather like an MOT test on a car: they are only really valid on the day they are carried out. One rather expensive way of attempting to offset this problem is to do a series of interviews, with the same people. However, a large number of qualitative studies only report 'one-off' interviews.

Third is the issue of the meaning we find in what other people say. As we listen to people or as we read transcriptions of what they have said, we develop what we imagine to be an understanding of their point of view. However, without constantly checking for understanding, it is impossible to know whether or not we have captured the particular meaning that the person in front of us is trying to convey. People use words in different ways and their understandings of the meanings of those words vary. In an interview, there are two people who are battling to understand each other's meaning systems. There is room, here, for considerable misunderstanding and error.

Questionnaires

The data that arises out of questionnaires is usually of a quantitative nature: respondents are asked to tick boxes or circle a response. These data are then summarised and presented either as numbers of items or as percentage responses. Sometimes, people who devise questionnaires also include some open questions, which allow the respondent to write a few words or sentences to express a view. These sections of a questionnaire are sometimes considered to produce 'qualitative' data but, in the end, responses to these questions are often very limited.

Where it *is* possible to obtain lengthier responses to open questions, that run to more than a few words or sentences, the data can be analysed in the same way as data obtained from interviews – as indicated above and in Chapter 11, which discusses qualitative data analysis in detail. Naturally, the element of interaction with an interviewer will be absent, and, in consequence, so will both the advantages and disadvantages of the qualitative interview.

Observation

In qualitative research, observation usually takes place under the heading of ethnographic studies. The research aims to note the everyday life of a small or large group of people. While the quantitative researcher is likely to have a list of behaviours to observe and 'tick off' or count, the qualitative one will be more interested in describing, as carefully as possible, what he or she sees. In the ethnographic style of research, no guidelines are developed to guide the researcher to what he or she is observing. Instead, the researcher takes a 'naturalistic' approach and keeps field notes about what he or she has observed that day.

The notes arising out of such research are bound to be impressionistic and cannot be claimed to be an accurate record of 'what is going on'. However, one of the tasks of the researcher is to *ask* the people whom he or she observes for explanations of their behaviour. Perhaps the most common area in which such observation is used is in *cultural* research, where the researcher is attempting to understand how different people lead ordinary lives in cultures other than their (the researcher's) own.

There is a particular problem here. On the one hand, the researcher wants to involve herself in what she is observing, in order to try to understand what she is observing. On the other hand, the researcher also wants to be able to 'stand back' a little, so that observation is possible. If the researcher is too close to those being observed, her report will be too subjective: her own presence is also likely to colour both the report and the behaviour being observed. On the other hand, if the researcher stands too far back from what she is observing, much observation will be lost: the researcher simply will not understand what is being observed.

Similarly, there is what may be known as the 'insider/outsider' problem when it comes to observation in different cultures. Those who are 'in' a culture may well not appreciate the significance of what they are doing or how their behaviour differs from that of other people, in other cultures. Thus, the researcher who is from the culture under observation may take many things for granted. However, the researcher who is from outside the culture may have problems, too. She may not even *notice* significant actions nor understand the meanings behind the behaviours being observed.

An example may be useful here. One of us recently completed a study about culture and communication in Thai healthcare. The study was an ethnographic one and involved both observation and interviews. The following example arises out of that study and demonstrates the issues of 'insider/outsider' understanding of culture.

Insider and outsider perspectives

When Thai people go out for a drink or for a meal – and they nearly always do this in a group – the most senior person pays the bill at the end of the evening. The seniority runs roughly along the lines of age, position, likely salary. Nothing has to be said: Thai people are always working out who, in any given situation, is 'senior' or 'junior' to them. The most senior person will, then, pick up the bill and it will be unremarkable. No one would expect to contribute to the payment.

Let us consider this from the points of view of the 'insider' (the Thai person, at the table) and from the point of view of the 'outsider' (a visitor from another culture). The Thai person is likely not even to notice how the bill gets paid. Nor, if he or she has not travelled, may he or she consider that this is anything different from what goes on in other cultures. In other words, the Thai person is likely to be blind to the significance of this piece of behaviour.

The person from another culture observing this situation – and without knowing about this particular sort of 'bill-paying' behaviour – may believe that (a) the person paying the bill has invited his friends out and is paying the bill as a goodwill gesture or that (b) the bill payer is simply a very generous person, who refuses to take payment from other people at the table. If either of these is the case, then the outsider will *also* be blind to the significance of the behaviour. The bill-paying episode will go by, not really noticed by either insider or outsider.

We suspect that many of these cultural behaviours take place that are both ignored by the insider and unnoticed by the outsider. For this reason, the ethnographic observer needs to be prepared to question a great deal of what he or she sees. There are limits to this. Out with friends, in Thailand, I was asked: 'why do you ask so many odd questions!' Clearly, it is important not become intrusive. In the Thai study, it also helped that both an outsider (PB) and an insider (a Thai researcher) conducted the work. In this way, the two could constantly compare their observations and challenge each other on the supposed 'meaning' of what was going on.

Field notes, then, are the notes collected from observations made in the field of study. They are best written as soon after a period of observation as possible (although, sometimes, a 'period of observation' can be a whole work shift or even a whole day). There is no particular formula for the writing of such notes. Alongside or included within these notes, it is often useful to include *descriptive* passages that define the *context* of observation. Thus, the researcher may report, in his or her notes, descriptions of the area in which he or she is working. Here is a short example of a field note from my Thai study.

Field notes

Bangkok. Seven in the morning. Outside, the city is spread out like a grubby tablecloth. To my right, the spaghetti junction of the flyovers, already thick with traffic. To my right, the 7-11 sign. We sat outside the 7-11 till late, last night, drinking and waiting for the rain to stop. Rangnam Road flooded as we sat there and we waded home with umbrellas.

The land outside is covered in concrete buildings. Much of it is of a type found all over South East Asia, smallish, two or three story, concrete buildings of a very utilitarian type. However, that landscape is also punctuated by very distinctive Thai buildings. Vegetation springs up in the cracks between. Down below my balcony is the tiny sub-soi that links us to Rangnam. There is so much green in Bangkok. An apple-head Siamese cat strolls down it. These are not the delicate, pointed faced, creatures that many people in Britain like and that win prizes in cat competitions. Rather, they are solid animals with big round faces. Cats round here spend a lot of time outside and seem to look after themselves, or, perhaps, neglect themselves. As do dogs. There are now so many feral dogs in Bangkok that monks in the *wats* are being asked to take them in. I suspect that the Buddhist culture prevents there from being a cull of these animals. Quite why the monks should have to have them, though, remains a mystery to me – perhaps because they do not feel they can refuse to. All around, birds are singing, still audible above the traffic noise. There is a cock crowing.

There are tightly packed living quarters everywhere that you can see. Tiny rooms with broken windows or bars up at the windows. A large palm tree sprouts next to someone's home and must block their light and their view. Last night, I watched a family group sitting in one of the tiny courtyards between the buildings. Mother and father were both carefully checking through their young daughter's hair for nits or lice.

The sun is already hot. It will rain again today and perhaps flood again. Most frequently, it first rains at almost the same hour every day: 4 pm.

In between the slum dwellings are tall, chunky apartment buildings and hotels. To the right is the Ratchaprop Tower Mansion, a Chinese place, probably, as it is also named in Chinese characters. Someone, to the left, has cultivated a room garden. Perhaps this is where the birds sing. There is lots of room for other roof gardens in this maze of unfinished buildings. Perhaps they will build on top of them, once the money comes back to Bangkok. If it ever does. I must check to see if there is a 'roof tax', in Thailand, as is the case in some other countries. If there is, then perhaps sometimes people leave the top parts of their houses unfinished.

In the distance, the taller, more elegant tower blocks of Saphan Kwai and north Bangkok. The city seems to go on forever.

The city is coming to life and is noisy. Immediately north of me, the elevated road is already chock full. Two more palms sit impassively underneath. 'KA', says a sign, 'The Symbolic of Beauty'. Or it might be, if I knew what the sign was for. This is a case of the semiotic problem of the 'signifier slipping away from the signified'. You have to know about the product, in the first place, to know what the advert is trying to persuade you to buy. In this case, a further complication lies in the sign being displayed in English. The billboard advert, then, appeals to English speaking people, who already know what the KA product is.

Bangkok is full of huge signs and billboards. They are part of the popular culture of the place.

Clearly, not all such notes will be used. The point, though, is to be as *inclusive* as possible in these notes. Decisions can be taken, at a later date, about what is finally kept and what is discarded (or, perhaps, kept for another report: it is often good to 'revisit' data and to re-analyse them in different ways).

Notes such as these can be analysed, using a form of content analysis that is described in Chapter 11. It may be noted that *any* type of text can be analysed and put into categories where each category represents a particular sort of issue. Although a huge literature has grown around the processes of analysing qualitative data, there is nothing too complicated in the process. Essentially, it consists of grouping passages of text together that are similar to each other.

Published work

A final possibility for collecting data exists in previously published work. Slightly different from a systematic review of the literature, here, the researcher looks for passages of text that support or refute the points that he or she is making in her study. Thus, following making the above field notes, I went to the literature to see what I could find on 'Bangkok bill posts' and came up with a great deal of information about the 'art' of such posters.

Another possibility, here, is a review of a particular set of journals or newspapers. It is possible to conduct 'thematic analyses' of such sets by searching for particular themes and issues. This form of analysis can also make use of what is sometimes called the 'template' approach. In most forms of qualitative data analysis, the researcher tries to identify naturally occurring themes. In the template approach, the researcher already has questions in mind to 'ask of the data'. For example, a researcher might search through a complete back-set of education journals to see what has been written about curriculum development. Then, using direct quotations from these journals, the researcher prepares a report that is not dissimilar to any other qualitative research report – examples of which can be found in the following chapter.

The type of evidence being produced from all these sorts of studies is important. It is not *quantified* evidence and we cannot, easily, generalise from it. However, findings from such studies can give us important insights into how to care for people from other cultures and what other people's views of healthcare are. I think I can say, with some certainty, that I understand the Thai culture a little better than I did five years ago. This is not to claim that I know everything about how Thai people live and work or even very much. Simply, though, I am more aware of the complexity of relationships between some Thai people. Interestingly, too, I have become more aware of my *own* culture, in the process. For if you study the culture of another group, you also take your own culture with you. A simple example, here, will suffice. Thai people, generally, do not say 'hello' and 'goodbye' or 'please' and 'thank you' very much (although the culture is a very polite one). By contrast, British people have usually been acculturated to the point where 'please' and 'thank you' are almost said too often – or, perhaps more typically, 'sorry'!

I remember worrying that I had upset a colleague in some way as he never said 'hello' to me on meeting – even if I had just arrived in the country. I asked other colleagues if this was the case and I was assured that: 'Everything is fine!' It was not until much later that I appreciated that the terms of greeting and parting are used so rarely. In fact, it could be taken as a sign that I had, to a small degree, become part of the group as people no-longer needed to do the very 'English' thing of saying 'hello'. The point, here, is that it is *useful* to know small details like this. This sort of evidence, when collected together, can make positive differences to the ways in which we care for other people, from different cultures. It is also the kind of fine grain examination of human experience which is at the heart of good qualitative data collection. In the following three chapters, we look at three particularly widely used approaches to putting that data collection into practice in qualitative research.

Review questions

Is qualitative research supposed to be representative? If not, how may it be useful?

What are the advantages and disadvantages of unstructured, semi-structured and structured interviews?

Might particular sampling approaches be better for some types of interview than others?

> **Exercise**
>
> Consider yourself as an insider and as an outsider. Write a brief list of words and behaviours which are particular to an insider group you belong to. Try to recall what it felt like before you became an insider.

Reference

Patton, M.Q. (1990) *Qualitative Evaluation and Research Methods*, 2nd edn. Newbury Park, CA: Sage.

Further reading

Burnard, P. (2005) *Counselling Skills for Health Professionals*, 4th edn. Gloucester: Nelson-Thornes.

Egan, G. (2002) *The Skilled Helper: A Problem-Management and Opportunity-Development Approach to Helping*, 7th edn. Pacific Grove: Brooks/Cole.

Gerrish, K. (1997) Being a 'marginal native': dilemmas of the participant observer. *Nurse Researcher*, 5(1), 25–34.

Kreuger, R.A. (1988). *Focus Groups: A Practical Guide for Applied Research*. London: Sage.

Krueger, R.A. and Mary, A.C. (2000). *Focus Groups: A Practical Guide for Applied Research*. Thousand Oaks, CA: Sage.

Kvale, S. (1996) *Interviews: An Introduction to Qualitative Research Interviewing*. Thousand Oaks, CA: Sage.

Newell, R. (1994) *Interviewing Skills for Nurses and Other Health Care Professionals: A Structured Approach*. London: Routledge.

Oppenheim, A.N. (1992) *Questionnaire Design, Interviewing and Attitude Measurement*, 2nd edn. London: Pinter.

Simmons, R. (1993) Questionnaires. In: N. Gilbert (ed.), *Researching Social Life*. London: Sage.

Stewart, D.W. and Shamdasani, P.N. (1992). *Focus Groups: Theory and Practice*. London: Sage.

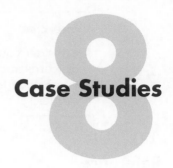

Case Studies

Introduction

Case studies are part of a particular style of descriptive, qualitative research. Descriptive research is that which seeks *only* to describe and inform (as opposed to testing a hypothesis or attempting prediction). The main value of such description, perhaps, is to 'illuminate' a situation, a culture or a group of people – sometimes, the case study approach is used to describe a single person's situation. The case study can make

Research for Evidence-Based Practice in Healthcare, Second edition, by Robert Newell and Philip Burnard
© 2011 Robert Newell and Philip Burnard

the reader think and allow him or her to ask questions such as 'does this study record things that are similar or different to my own experience' and 'what can I use from this study to inform my own practice'.

What remains clear is that anyone using the qualitative, case study approach should never be tempted to generalise from such work. It is tempting, at the end of any research report, to offer recommendations – either general recommendations or ones specifically for practice. The researcher who offers case studies, however, can only ever say (in so many words): 'Look! This is what I found and this is what happened in one situation, at one time in history: make of it what you will!' Given that case studies are only usually about a small number of people, a specific situation or place, the 'findings' that are reported can never be generalised out to larger populations. It is the case that another researcher, on another day, may have described things differently. Similarly, on another day, the situation, itself, might have been different. People and places change over time. The case study can only ever offer a glimpse of what life was like for a limited number of people, in a very particular place at a very specific time. Naturally, this can be an extremely useful insight in itself, and may guide practice if one's circumstances are similar to those of the case study situation.

Case studies can be used in at least two ways. First, they can be used as 'illustrations' in a larger study. Second, they can be used as the main data collection, analysis and reporting method. Both approaches are now elaborated.

The case study as 'illustration'

In qualitative research – and particularly, perhaps, in ethnography (which is described in the next chapter) – the researcher often finds that one of his or her respondents or one of the places he visits rewards him or her with considerably more – or more detailed – data. For example, a particular interviewee may be able to answer questions in considerably greater depth than his colleagues or a college that is visited is more 'open' to the researcher. In these cases, it is sometimes useful to use such 'outstanding' sets of data in the form of a case study. Such a case study may offer a more detailed account of the principle being – more generally – described by the researcher in his or her presentation of findings.

However, a caveat needs to be added here. Very often (unless the researcher has planned a particular case study, in advance), the material used in a case-study-as-illustration, will not be typical of the points under discussion. The person, for example, who offers a very in-depth interview, may be more extrovert than a number of his colleagues or, perhaps, have very strong views on the topic in hand. Thus, it becomes important *not* simply to offer a case study, using this material, as a 'typical example' of what is being discussed. The case study must be presented *only* as a single example of a person's or place's situation. Indeed, the researcher may want to highlight, in his or her text, the ways in which this case study differs from the other data being presented or, of course, the ways in which it is similar. Always, as we have noted, the researcher must resist any temptation to generalise from a case study and resist making suggestions as to how others might change their practice as a result of reading the case study. It must be emphasised that the case study can only offer one illustration of a given but specific situation.

The point just made might usefully be made about *all* qualitative research. Qualitative research is useful in illustrating and describing. It can help offer a particular and sometimes historical view of people, places and things. However, it is never safe to generalise from qualitative findings. Even if findings appear to 'replicate' the findings of another study, they do not. The sampling and analysis methods used in qualitative research make this impossible. An apparent 'replication study' is not really any such thing: it is quite possibly coincidence at work if a researcher's findings are very similar to another's.

The case-study-as-illustration, within a larger study, can be developed in a variety of ways. First, the case study can be a boxed section, within the findings section of the study and, rather literally, serve as an illustration. The main body of the text will refer the reader to this boxed section and thus point to it as an in-depth example of what he or she found. The account, within the box, will often contain a descriptive passage about the person(s) involved or the place being described. It will then give an account of what happened and of the outcome of the described events. When the case study is drawn from an interview, it is possible to present the data verbatim. Thus, the boxed section will contain a short transcript of the interview and report both the interviewer *and* the interviewee's words. Those words may or may not be followed by a short discussion of the transcription – perhaps relating it back to the body of the research report.

Second, the case study can be offered as a separate section within a research report. This allows the researcher more space to develop an in-depth account of a specific place, person or event. However, it is normally the case that reporting qualitative findings takes up a lot of words. The researcher should bear in mind that most research is usually reported (in published format) in journals. This means that the research has to be extremely economical with words. The student who completes a dissertation or thesis may want to include the case study in *that* research report but choose not to use it in a paper submitted to a journal. Alternatively, he or she may choose to publish the case study as a separate paper.

Third, the case study within a research report can be the result of a planned activity. The researcher might decide, for example, to interview one or two respondents in greater depth than would be the case with others. In this way, he or she plans, in advance, the nature of his or her case study material. The researcher may draw up a specific pro forma to enable him or her to collect data in a relatively systematic way. Such a pro forma may contain background and/or biographical information about each case study subject, followed by the respondents' views and ideas. In doing this, the researcher stands to present uniform case studies, both in terms of length and layout.

The case study as a research method

The alternative position is for the researcher to use the case study method as the main research method in a particular study. Here, a decision will have been made to describe, in considerable detail, a particular person, group of people, place or object. For example, a midwife, in considering the experience of pregnancy, may follow the experience of one or more pregnant women through their pregnancies. He or she may ask that person or persons to keep diaries of their thoughts, feelings and actions, interview them at regular intervals and ask for further interviews after the birth of the baby.

As is often the case in qualitative research, the researcher may use lesser or greater structure in the collection of data. The midwife, for example, in advising pregnant women about keeping diaries may (a) offer them a format for recording their thoughts, feelings and actions or (b) simply ask them to regularly 'write in your diary'. These two approaches are likely to yield different sorts of findings. Data collected from the more structured approach are likely to be easier to analyse, whilst 'freeform' data are often very difficult to categorise and report. However, the amount and depth of the data obtained may be much greater in the second approach.

Similarly, interviews can range from 'very structured' – in which case the data collection method can become almost the use of a 'verbal questionnaire' – to totally unstructured (in which the researcher has no previously worked out agenda for the interview and opens it with a very broad, open question such as 'I am interested in anything you can tell me about your thoughts on X' [where 'X' is the topic focused on in the study]). Again, the same pros and cons apply. Very tightly structured interviews are less likely to yield rich or in-depth data, but are likely to be easier to analyse. Totally unstructured interviews are likely to reveal different and often idiosyncratic findings but are likely to be difficult to categorise and analyse.

Depending on the amount of autonomy that the researcher can exercise, it is possible to supplement case studies in various ways. For example, the researcher may want to include photographs or even sound track material to further illuminate the case study material. These approaches can offer a more three-dimensional picture within the case study. However, it is impossible to know how the consumer of such a report is going to respond to seeing photographs or hearing sounds. It might be felt that such an approach further adds to the subjectivity of the report. It might be borne in mind, however, that many other forms of reporting about other people, *do* include illustrations: travel writing and journalism are frequently supplemented in this way and such illustrations serve to 'personalise' the reporting. A topic for consideration is, indeed, the degree to which some forms of qualitative research (and case study) differ from, or are similar to, travel writing and journalism. Both media seek to report 'honestly' about their subject matter (as does qualitative research). Both often offer historical, theoretical or political background information about the topic or place under discussion – again, as is the case in qualitative research reporting. Finally, in both journalism and qualitative research, the author/researcher recognises their role within the situation they are examining and reporting on, and does not seek to be remote or objective in the way which is often associated with quantitative research. Their role in the research and reporting is seen as a valid contribution to our understanding. One important difference, perhaps, is that travel writers – in particular – are, presumably, seeking to entertain as well as inform their readers. Researchers, on the other hand, should, presumably, be dedicated to reporting, as closely as possible, 'things as they are' or, at least, 'things as they appear to be' – regardless of whether or not their research writing is in any sense entertaining.

Drawbacks

There are, of course, some drawbacks with the case study approach – whether it is of the illustrative sort of the 'stand-alone' variety. If, for example, the researcher depends upon one person to supply the data for a case study, there is a danger that the person may (a) withdraw from the study, (b) default on recording data, (c) move from the district, or even (d) die. If any of these things happen, then the research is put in jeopardy.

Choosing a sample – either in terms of a person, persons or place(s) can also be difficult. People agreeing to be the single focus of a research study may not be typical of the group to which they belong. Similarly, focusing on one organisation or one place will inevitably lead to comparisons between that organisation or place and others. I (PB) found this a particular problem when describing Thai healthcare education (in an ethnographic study). I realised that it was almost impossible to describe that system without, at the same time, comparing it to the UK or American system of education. This *may* not necessarily be a problem, but it *can* lead to a debate about the 'rightness' or 'wrongness' of a given system. Such value judgements often fall in favour of the system from which the researcher is reporting. The challenge, then, in case studies, is to attempt to describe a single person, place, event or thing, without too much comparison with others. The point is, perhaps, to describe, describe, describe and attempt to offer very little analysis or value judgement. However, in reality, such a task is difficult to attempt and even less likely to be an achievable outcome.

A further problem is that, at the outset, the single-person study might appear to be an interesting one that will yield considerable, in depth, data. However, the reality might be that such data is not gleaned and that it becomes difficult to justify the reporting of a story that turns out to be fairly shallow or monotonous. This is not to suggest the other people's lives are necessarily boring but to highlight the fact that the case study approach *may* not answer the initial research question. It may be the case that the case study exploration turns out to produce little that is exploratory.

A further possible problem with the single-case-study approach (in the qualitative style) is the degree to which other researchers (and publishers) accept it as a valid form or research. If some of them do not, it may be difficult to have the final work published. Perhaps the most extreme version of the single-case-study approach, which both of us have come across, was a study in which the researcher used himself as the focus of study. The research report consisted of a reporting of that person's own views and thoughts. The idea of such an enterprise raises considerable questions about our own ability to stand back from ourselves and, in any real sense, report accurately and objectively what we are researching. On the other hand, some might claim that qualitative research – and particularly the case study approach – lacks objectivity, anyway. Thus, the 'researcher as focus for study' might be acceptable. On balance, though, it is safe to say that such an approach does not, as yet, have universal appeal as a research method in healthcare and the neophyte researcher might be well advised not to use it. Generally, careful thought should be given to the selection of any method of data collection and analysis and the limitations of the case study approach should not be underestimated.

It should be noted that, sometimes, the term 'case study' is used to refer to a study of a single *organisation* (see Cooke, 2006, for an example of a case study of three NHS institutions using multiple data collection approaches). In this approach, a range of methods are used, including interviews, observation and the study of organisational documentation. In this way, a picture of the entire organisation is built up. Another term that has been used for this approach is *illuminative evaluation*. This form of evaluation is usually used in the study of a school or other educational institution. Its aim, as it suggests, is to illuminate the workings of the organisation, from all angles: from the students', from the teachers', from the managers' and from the point of view of any other stakeholders.

To what degree might the case study approach be said to add to the 'evidence base' of evidence-based healthcare? Certainly, as we have seen, the findings from any form of qualitative study cannot be generalised to larger populations[1]. We have also noted, however, that qualitative studies – and, perhaps, in particular, the case study, can have *illuminative* qualities. Case studies can show healthcare workers a particular view of what happens in medicine and healthcare. This they can do in a similar way to the use of pictures in books. The case study is often a graphic and easily understood way of capturing a particular moment in history and in a particular context.

Review questions

Is it ever possible to generalise from case studies?
In what two main ways can case studies be used? Do these different forms of use lead to different ways of interpreting the data?
How problematic are the main drawbacks of case studies?

Exercise

Imagine you were going to mount a case study in an organisation of which you are a member (e.g., your place of work, your university or a hobby group). Make a brief note of what sort of data would tell you most about how that organisation functions, and how you would go about collecting it. Consider how your choice of data collection might (or might not) lead to a biased picture of the organisation.

Endnote

1. Some would argue that if a range of qualitative studies report very similar things, then those findings might, carefully, be aggregated and carefully generalised. We believe that this is to pile error upon error. If it is not possible to generalise from *one* study, then bringing together a range of studies (from which generalisation is not possible) does not strengthen the position from which to generalise.

Reference

Cooke, H.F. (2006) The surveillance of nursing standards: an organisational case study. *International Journal of Nursing Studies*, 43, 975–984.

Further reading

Darker, P., Shanks, G. and Broadbent, M. (1998) Successfully completing case study research: Combining rigour, relevance and pragmatism. *Information Systems Journal*, 8, 273–289.

Merriman, S.B. (1988) *Case Study Research in Education: A Qualitative Approach*. San Francisco: Jossey-Bass.

Stake, R.E. (1995) *The Art of Case Study Research*. Thousand Oaks, CA: Sage.

Yin, R.K. (1993) *Applications of Case Study Research*. Newbury Park, CA: Sage.

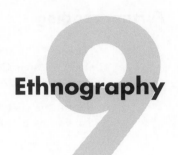

Ethnography

Introduction

Ethnography is a qualitative approach to research. Traditionally, it involves the in-depth study of a culture. The term 'culture' refers to the

Research for Evidence-Based Practice in Healthcare, Second edition, by Robert Newell and Philip Burnard
© 2011 Robert Newell and Philip Burnard

ways in which people live together, their behaviours, thoughts, feelings, beliefs and ways of doing things. In the past, ethnographic research tended to investigate cultures that were very different from that of the researcher. For example, an ethnographer might live for a time in a distant country, meet and talk to the people, observe them in everyday life and then write a detailed report of his or her findings. Increasingly, the ethnographic approach has grown to include studying cultural aspects of everyday life in the researcher's own culture and studying the 'culture' or organisations or specific groups of people. For example, a researcher might use an ethnographic approach in studying how people cope after major surgery. This would be a kind of sub-culture consisting of recovering patients[1].

Previously, instructions on the methods used in ethnographic research were few. Students of ethnography would be told simply to go out into a culture and look at what happened there and then write their report. Increasingly, as is the case with other forms of qualitative research, methods have tended to become more focused and specific.

It sometimes helps to distinguish between *ethnography* and *ethnographic methods*. An ethnography usually arises in the fields of anthropology or sociology and is the 'classic' form, described in the first paragraph. As we have noted, the ethnographer might live in a distant country and write a book about his or her experiences and observations. Ethnographic methods, on the other hand, while drawing on the traditional ethnographic approach, may refer to interviews and observations made in other contexts and, sometimes, used in combination with other forms of research methods. In the latter case, the term 'mixed method research' is sometimes used.

The stages of an ethnographic study

Organising an ethnographic study takes time but that organisation follows similar principles to any other research. First, the researcher must identify the question that he or she is seeking to answer. As is the case with other forms of research, inexperienced researchers tend to ask questions that are too large and all-encompassing and it is important to work with a supervisor who can help make the question more focused and particular. This can be especially problematic with ethnography, as, by their very nature, the sorts of topics addressed are already very broad.

Second, the researcher has to learn or rehearse the methods of data collection and data analysis that are to be used. Often, doing ethnographic research is a 'one-off' process. It is rarely possible to return to respondents (or even places) to clarify issues that have not been covered in the original encounter. If this *is* possible, then so much the better. As the ideal, it is good to take an iterative approach to data collection.

That is to say that the researcher meets respondents (or goes to places) on many occasions, in order to deepen an understanding of the culture or to clarify data that have been collected previously. In practice, however, most researchers have neither the time nor the funds to do this. They need, therefore, to be confident in using data collection methods that will obtain the right data and in sufficient quantities.

Third, arrangements have to be made to access the field of study. This may involve complex practicalities such as buying plane or train tickets, booking accommodation, agreeing leave. It may also involve having the research proposal checked and agreed by one or more ethics committees. While not all countries have ethics committees, many – if the researcher wants to access patients or healthcare workers – do. Clearly, adjustments may have to be made to a proposal in the light of an ethics committee decision and there is always the possibility that a proposal may be rejected by such a committee.

The issue of having to obtain ethical approval and also of obtaining informed consent from informants may add a problem to the research plan. If the researcher wants to collect 'naturalistic' data – data about ordinary people, doing ordinary things in a 'natural' rather than controlled environment, the fact of their knowing that research on them is taking place may alter their behaviour. Thus, the resulting study is not one of 'natural observation' but 'observation of people who know they are being studied'. In the end, there is no easy answer to this issue. It is right and proper that ethical approval and consent to take part in a study are obtained and these two take precedent over the 'authenticity' of the study. Clearly, however, there are instances where it is impossible to get consent (e.g., in an observational study of risky behaviour in crowds, it would be impractical to seek consent from every member of a football audience). By the same token, in such situations the degree of intrusion into an individual's life is trivial, and so the need for their consent is thereby diminished.

Fourth, the researcher has to move into the field. This means making personal adjustments to life in a different place and a different culture, and this can be as true of researching in an unfamiliar culture in one's own country (say, amongst homeless intravenous drug users) as in the more obviously different environment of an overseas study. At first, everything seems new and different. This can be both a good and a bad thing. The good thing is that the researcher arrives with 'fresh eyes' and notices all those things that might be lost to a person who was native to that culture. The bad thing is that all this new input may daze the researcher and he or she may be unsure either what to note and record or what it all means. This is sometimes called 'ethnographic dazzle'. In the author's experience, it is surprising how quickly this initial phase passes and the 'strange' becomes 'ordinary'. Everyone wants to fit in and become comfortable in the place they are living – even if they are living there only temporarily. As a result, we probably try to accept what is going on very quickly. Again, this is both good and bad news for the ethnographic researcher. On the one hand, he or she quickly adapts to cultural differences. On the other hand, a considerable amount of cultural sensitivity may be lost in the process. The researcher may, fairly quickly, take for granted that which he or she observes. Added to this is the possibility that the researcher's taken-for-granted view of what he or she observes may be erroneous – in the understandable rush that he or she has to 'fit in'.

Fifth, the researcher needs to collect data and the methods used for this are described below – as are the methods used to analyse and report on those data.

Finally, the researcher removes him or herself from the field and is free to ponder on the experiences that have been observed. Again, there are positive and negative elements to this withdrawal. Being distanced from the field allows time for reflection and consideration of the data. However, the very fact of being out of the culture may mean that erroneous conclusions are drawn from that data. It is very easy to theorise about culture when the person is many miles away from it. There may also be little opportunity for 'fact checking' with a person or a respondent from the culture that has been observed. Consideration should always be made, in initial planning, to make sure, where at all possible, that such contacts *are* available. We have found that the best solution to this problem is, when possible, to undertake joint research with a person who is native to the culture under consideration. This may mean linking with a colleague who is an HCP, a researcher, or simply someone who lives in the culture.

Stages in an ethnographic study

Identify question
Learn or rehearse data collection methods (ethnography is often 'one-off')
Arrange access (including practicalities)
Enter the field
Collect data
Leave the field and reflect

General methods used in ethnographic research

The aim of ethnographic research, as we have seen, is to capture something of another culture. Thus, the ethnographer or ethnographic researcher uses his or her senses to capture aspects of that culture. A summary of the methods used in this approach is now described.

Everyday observation is one of the major methods. The ethnographer lives in the chosen setting, observes what is going on and keeps detailed 'fieldnotes'. He or she has constantly to question what is being observed. It is a fact that we carry our own culture with us at all times and tend, if we are not careful, to compare and contrast everything we see with our own cultural beliefs and our own learned behaviour. Thus, we may erroneously draw conclusions about what we see in a different culture, based on our own background. The skilled ethnographer, then, tries hard to see things afresh and simply to act as a detached observer, while, at the same time, living amongst the people whom he or she is observing. Clearly, this is no easy task. The accent, in ethnographic research is on 'normal', everyday behaviour: the ethnographer is seeking to describe (and later, perhaps, to explain) how ordinary people, in different cultures, live their lives.

Alongside observation, the ethnographer talks to people and tries to get them to explain aspects of their culture. This is done through interview, conversation and even through chance encounters on an everyday basis. The point, again, is not simply to compare and contrast what others do with the cultural background of the researcher but to attempt to describe what is going on, in the culture's *own* terms. Again, this is not an easy thing to achieve. It is easy for the ethnographer to draw the wrong conclusions based on his or her own lack of understanding of the 'different' culture. Similarly, the person who 'in' the other culture may not question his or her own practices nor even know *why* he or she does something in a particular way. We are all, to a small or large extent, blind to our own culture.

An example, here, may help and it is drawn from my own (PB) experience of doing ethnographic research, in healthcare communication, in Thailand.

In Thailand, when people go out for a meal, it is standard practice for the most senior person at the table to pay the bill. This is also true for friends or colleagues going out for a drink in a bar (in Thai bars, all drinks are paid for when people leave the bar and not on a pay-as-you-go basis as is the case in some countries – including the UK). The senior and junior issue, in Thailand, is an important one and all Thais are able to assess, very quickly, who is senior and who is junior to them. This, broadly, can be identified in terms of the other person's age, their relative wealth, their job title, but also in a range of other, more subtle ways. Suffice to say that Thai people do not usually make mistakes in these distinctions.

This senior–junior ranking, although it happens, is not so clear-cut in Northern European or American countries. So, let us consider a Northern European person observing the end of a meal at a restaurant in Thailand. He or she observes that one person picks up the bill for all of those present. That person does not suggest a sharing of the bill and no one else at the table makes such an offer. The bill is received and paid quickly. To the Thai person, this is not remarkable and would neither be commented on or thought about. It just happens. However, to the Northern European observer, a variety of 'wrong' conclusions may be drawn. First, he or she might think that the person who paid the bill had invited all the other guests for a meal. Second, he or she might imagine that the person who paid was 'generous'. Third, he or she may believe that the person paying the bill is in some way 'returning the compliment' and choosing to pay, having been at previous meals where others paid. Without cultural insight, that observer is very unlikely to appreciate the 'real' reason behind this action. Thus, the observer is 'blind' to an aspect of culture, while the Thai guests think nothing of it. If this meal was to be part of an ethnographic study, an important aspect of Thai culture might be lost.

The ethnographic researcher, then, has constantly to challenge the ordinary and to be prepared to ask the questions: 'why does that happen?', 'how did that happen?' or 'what does that mean?' Those questions must be addressed both, internally, to the researcher him or herself and to those he or she observes or talks to. This often involves great tact and diplomacy. The author recalls being asked, by a group of friends, in Thai bar: 'why do you ask so many strange questions?'

Interviews, in ethnographic research, need to be recorded. While this is normally done with the aid of a tape recorder, as noted in Chapter 7, this may not be practical in natural, informal settings, in which case very detailed notes are an important substitute.

Consideration needs to be given to the storing of data when the researcher is in the field. This may be done through the use of notebooks, or – better – through the use of a laptop computer. If the former method is used, notebooks must be safely stored and if the later method is used, regular back-ups to a CD ROM or a USB portable storage device should be made. Another safety measure is to e-mail data files to yourself, the researcher. On returning home, the data are then safely stored in your e-mail account.

Fieldnotes should be kept. It is useful to complete these, where possible, at the same time, every day. Time should be set aside to type up an account of what has been observed and what has been done during the day. These notes can include tentative theories about what has been observed and include useful reference material. As is always the case, references to papers and research should be very carefully recorded so that those references can lead directly to the papers themselves.

Notes, on computer, can either be stored in word-processing files or by using a freeform database such as *askSam* or *OneNote*. While most database programs are highly structured in their layout, these programs allow you to store notes of any length, each as separate 'cards' in the database system. Particular pages can then be found or the entire database can be searched using keywords or Boolean operators (e.g. undertaking searches such as 'Stress NOT physiotherapist', will identify pages that contain information about stress but not pages that include the terms 'stress' and 'physiotherapist'. Other operators can also be used). These freeform database programs serve as useful containers for large amounts of textual information, linked to a particular project. They can also contain photos, graphics and other forms of computer data – including pages from the internet.

As we have noted, it is useful to make notes about ideas and theories as the research project unfolds. However, as with all theorising, it is best to keep theory to the absolute minimum and to proceed with great caution in developing those theories. The more elaborate the theory, the more likely it is to be wrong. It is often tempting to feel: 'I understand why that is happening!' but it is also vital to look for what can be called *disconfirming evidence*. In other words, as a potential theory emerges from the data, the researcher must always be asking: 'Could I be wrong?' and search for evidence that confounds the theory. In many cases, searching in this way will lead the researcher to question the appropriateness or 'fit' of the theory.

What should be observed?

This is a question that often baffles the first time ethnographic researcher. Much will depend upon how clearly the initial research question has been articulated. A clear question can direct the researcher to make fairly specific observations (by 'observations', in this context, we mean: 'what should be observed and what should be talked and asked about?') On the other hand, by its nature ethnography is concerned with the description of culture and this is, necessarily, often wide ranging. Many ordinary and everyday events can easily impinge on a wide range of (for example) healthcare practices.

A metaphor that may serve to help in this debate is that of a camera. Sometimes, the photographer will want a broad, landscape shot of a scene. At other times, he or she will want to zoom in on a detail, thus leaving out much of the background information. Similarly, the ethnographic researcher might want to work on two levels. First, he or she should remain open to observing very general, everyday practices within the culture under observation. Thus, fieldnotes might include details of a trip to the supermarket as well as the layout of hospital wards. Both of these areas are part of people's everyday, cultural experience.

However, he or she should be prepared, very quickly, to home in on particular, focused situations. What, for example, does an occupational therapist do when he or she talks to a patient about going home? What does he or she say? Where does he or she choose to speak to the patient? How does the patient respond? And then the researcher may choose to 'pan out' to the larger picture. How does this sort of episode fit into the broader life of the ward, the hospital and the community?

Another aid to considering what to observe is through the use of the idea of *rules*. Arguably, nations, communities, families and even individuals are governed by rules. There are written and unwritten rules for just about everything. There are, for example, rules about how to behave at funerals that are quite different from the rules governing weddings. There are rules about how to be a student radiographer as well as rules about how to be a radiography lecturer. There are rules about living with another person and about living in a street and in a town. The effective ethnographic researcher can often structure his or her observation by fairly frequently asking the question – in any context – 'what are the rules at work here?' This is a variant on the questions: 'why does this happen?' and 'what is going on here?' Attempting to codify or record the rules governing the way in which people work and live together, in this particular context, at this particular time, is often a fruitful way to proceed in ethnographic research.

Analysis

Once back home, the ethnographer is charged with analysing the data and organising it into readable passages of text. Perhaps the most usual way of doing this is to employ a form of *content analysis* – an umbrella term for a range of ways of organising textual data. Examples of how to do this are elaborated in Chapter 11, which explores qualitative data analysis in detail.

Once the data have been analysed, the (almost) final stage of the process is to write the research report (the final stage of any research project being the publication of findings in a journal or as a book). There are various styles of reporting. Some ethnographic accounts leave out details of previous literature and even of the methods used to collect and analyse the data. Most recently, however, the tendency has been for ethnographers to report their findings, more formally, in the style adopted by most other researchers.

As is the case with other types of qualitative research, there are two options in writing up the findings. One is to link the new findings from the study with other people's research and theories. The other is to present only the findings of the new study and relate them to other research only in the discussion. Here are two examples. The first is a reporting (of a fictitious project), with references to other people's work. The second is 'straight' reporting.

Reporting of findings related to other research

Many of the nurses who worked in Westland Hospital felt that they were isolated because the hospital was so far from the nearest town. While many chose to use the local bus service, some found themselves living what one called 'a very narrow and unexciting life'. This echoes the work done by Chalmers and Brown (2004), who studied the histories of mental hospitals in the UK and found that many staff felt that they had become 'institutionalised'. One nurse, in the present study, who had lived in at Westland for three years as a student and then found accommodation very close to it, had this to say:

'I find it hard to motivate myself to go out, sometimes. Well, I know I should! I know it's not healthy! But where would I go? Sometimes people say to me: "you should go to the movies or go clubbing in Eastland! But it's easy for them. Living here has made me feel that I've got nothing to talk about to anyone – even if I did go clubbing and stuff. It's difficult really"'.

Davies and Maddison (2003a, 2003b) identified, in staff in an isolated government post in North East Scotland, the problems of living close to the job and the feeling of 'not having anything to talk about'. The present study seems to add some confirmation to this being an issue of living so close to work. In their study, Davies and Maddison suggest:

'Living with the people you work with seems hardly healthy. Most people, it would seem, need to be able to make some division between work life and social life – although, we acknowledge that, in certain professions, this is not possible. It seems that this blurring of boundaries between home and professional life is viewed as "more acceptable" in those jobs were the employee has considerable autonomy in his or her work. It is, perhaps, less acceptable for those who do fairly routine work'. (Davies and Maddison, 2003a)

Reporting of findings not related to other research

Many of the nurses who worked in Westland Hospital felt that they were isolated because the hospital was so far from the nearest town. While many chose to use the local bus service, some found themselves living what one called 'a very narrow and unexciting life'. One nurse, in the present study, who had lived in at Westland for three years as a student and then found accommodation very close to it, had this to say:

'I find it hard to motivate myself to go out, sometimes. Well, I know I should! I know it's not healthy! But where would I go? Sometimes people say to me: "you should go to the movies or go clubbing in Eastland! But it's easy for them. Living here has made me feel that I've got nothing to talk about to anyone – even if I did go clubbing and stuff. It's difficult really"'.

> This feeling was often expressed, in the evenings, when nurses got together to chat over a drink in the Staff Club. Many of the conversations in the Club were about work – even if these were to complain about the conditions that led them to talk about work in the first place! A senior staff nurse, in the Club, said:
>
> 'It can't be good you. I have been on B6 for four years and most of the other nurses have been there for three or four. It's a funny place and we get on most of the time but we can get on each other's nerves. I get sick of talking about work all the time but we always seem to be at it! I suppose we are now really!'

Material from other research, like the findings of Brown and Chalmers (2004) and Davies and Maddison (2003a, 2003b), would then be reported separately in a discussion section and tied to the findings with a sentence of two.

Ethnographic reports, in full, are usually lengthy documents. The ethnographic researcher has to bear in mind many factors when deciding what to include and what to leave out of a report. The key issues are: for whom is the report being written? Is there a word limit? If the report is being written for submission as a PhD thesis, then it may include almost all the data that have been collected. Similarly, if it is being written as a book, it may also include most of the data but the style of the writing is likely to be more relaxed and less academic. Indeed, an interesting point for discussion might be the differences that do or do not exist between good travel writing and the writing of an ethnography. On the one hand, we might argue that travel writing undertaken as a means of entertaining (as well as informing) the reader. On the other hand, we might note that few ethnographers would want to produce totally uninteresting accounts!

If the ethnographic report is being written in the form of a paper for publication in a journal, other considerations have to be made. Normally, only part of the literature review will be reported and only a summary of the data collection and analysis methods recorded. Also, the researcher will have to make serious decisions about what findings to put in the report and what to leave out. These decisions can have serious consequences for the fidelity of the ethnographic account to the culture it attempts to portray. One approach to this latter issue is to consider writing a series of papers from the study, each of which reports different sets of data and thus each reporting a different aspect of the study.

Ethnography, like other qualitative methods, offers both the general reader and fellow researchers an illuminating and descriptive account of the area under study. Above all, it should be as faithful and as honest an account of what the research did and saw as possible, and it should help the reader to become acquainted with part of the world that, before, was something of a mystery.

From an evidence-based healthcare point of view, ethnographies can remind us of the importance of cultural context. We do not live in cultural isolation. We are surrounded by those who see the world differently from ourselves and who, in many ways, inhabit different worlds. The ethnography is a potent method of illustrating both the importance of culture and, with varying levels of success, how cultures 'work'.

Review questions

What, in your view, is the principal aim of ethnography?
What are the basic stages in undertaking an ethnographic study?
What are the chief advantages and drawbacks of immersion in a
    culture?

Exercise

Arrange to spend a morning in any unfamiliar subculture. It need not (and perhaps should not) be work related. For example, spend a day at an art gallery or in a bakery. Simply observe the goings on, the interactions, the formal and informal rules which make the setting work. This is the culture. How is it different from your own professional and personal subcultures.

Endnote

1. Perhaps *the* classic ethnographic study, which has been cited over and over again in healthcare, remains Erving Goffman's participant observation study *Asylums*, which describes the culture of total institutions. If you are familiar with this seminal work, you will probably see echoes of it in our fictionalised example of the staff of Westland Hospital. If you are not familiar with *Asylums*, or know it only through its many synopses and commentaries, or from lectures, we recommend strongly you read it in its original form, both because if its implications for healthcare (and not just in mental healthcare!), and as an example of intensive, sensitive research and reporting in ethnography.

Further reading

Agrosino, M. (2007) *Doing Ethnographic and Observational Research*. London: Sage.

Denzin, N.K. (1997) *Interpretive Ethnography: Ethnographic Practices for the 21st Century*. Thousand Oaks, CA: Sage.

Goffman, E. (1961) *Asylums: Essays on the Social Situation of Mental Patients and Other Inmates*. New York: Doubleday.

Hammersley, M. (1992) *What's Wrong with Ethnography*. London: Routledge.

Hine, C. (2000) *Virtual Ethnography*. Thousand Oaks, CA: Sage.

Le Compte, M.D., Preissle, J. and Tesch, R. (1993) *Ethnography and Qualitative Design in Educational Research*. San Diego: Academic Press.

McLachlan, M. (1997) *Culture and Health*. London: Wiley.

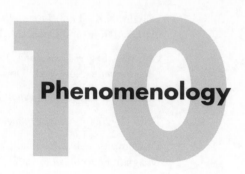

Phenomenology

Introduction

Phenomenological research, although distinctive, shares much in common with other approaches to qualitative research. This chapter explores some of the issues to do with understanding the phenomenological approach and also highlights ways in which it shares features with other approaches.

Research for Evidence-Based Practice in Healthcare, Second edition, by Robert Newell and Philip Burnard
© 2011 Robert Newell and Philip Burnard

Phenomenological research is concerned with how an *individual* views the world and how he or she lives his life – from *inside*. While many approaches to research look for commonalities of human experience (quantitative approaches, in particular, look for these), phenomenological research considers what it may be like to be *this* person, living *this* life at *this* time.

As I write these words, I (PB) do so from an office on the fourth floor of a small tower block. I can look away from the computer and out at more office buildings, two roads, a pedestrian walkway and at various trees. I can also look at a considerable expanse of sky. Presumably, further along the building, other colleagues can look out at the same or similar view. In one way, it is would not be difficult to identify the various elements of the scene, as it is viewed by a number of people. A photograph, taken from the window, would illustrate, very literally, the way things look outside the window on this particular day.

However, there is also a very different way to think about this. When I look out of the window, I also *respond* to what I see and these responses are likely to be different, for me, than they would be for a colleague in the next office. Let us consider some examples of this 'difference', for it is this 'lived experience' that is of interest to those doing phenomenological experience.

First, the trees, in summer, remind me of when I lived in Surrey, England (I now live in South Wales). A moment's glance brings back a whole range of memories of the past. Second, the buildings outside were built in the early 1970s and I have particular views about what has come to be called this 'brutalist' form of architecture. I am fascinated by the fact that once, in the 60s and 70s, I thought such buildings to be 'modern' and even beautiful and that now – along with many other people – I find them soulless and unattractive. One building reminds me of a hotel where I stay in Bangkok, Thailand – although, to anyone else, the association would, presumably, be a strange one. Third, I particularly enjoy watching a considerable number of seagulls flying and walking in the area. Two gulls, in particular, return year after year to mate and duly have a single, brown chick which, in turn, gets taught to become independent and fend for itself. All this reminds me of when I lived by the sea. Fourth, the sun on this scene can change my mood, just as a wet, dark day can.

In case it is not obvious, the scene is not in any sense a particularly memorable one. It is an ordinary, urban scene that exists, in a variety of forms, in cities in countries throughout the world. The point, here, of course, is that – in this case – *I* am looking at it! That, too, is unremarkable. But what is of interest is that at any time, in any given situation, *individuals* are looking at the world around them and feeling, thinking and even seeing, different things. They are making different associations, interpreting what they see in different ways and making judgments about what it is they look at.

If quantitative research (and, in some cases, ethnography) looks for similarities in the human condition, phenomenological research is concerned with the human, subjective experience. We can say about people that (a) they are similar, in ways, to all other people, (b) they are similar, in ways, to some other people, and that (c) they are, in ways, different from all other people. For example, I share, with all other people, certain physical characteristics: I have arms, legs, a head and so on. I probably share many of the worries I have with all other people: money concerns, worries about relationships and the like. I am also similar to some other people and not others. I am, for example, male, while some others are female. I am English, where others are from other countries and cultures. Finally, there are those things that are peculiar to me. These are probably mostly thoughts, feelings and beliefs. They are the odd quirks that make a person different. I happen to believe that the notion that everyone is unique is overstated. It seems likely, though, that there are peculiarities about us that are not shared by others. It should be noted, in passing, that if this 'unique element', this peculiarity that makes me, 'me' and which, in your case, makes you, 'you', how might we convey it to others?

Out of all this, then, the phenomenological researcher looks not for similarities but for the 'lived experience' of individual human beings. That researcher is looking for the subjective view, the view from the person who is peering out of the seemingly ordinary body. Again, a moment's reflection is likely to indicate that while we have a 'public' image, that we project both consciously and unconsciously, to others, we also have an 'private', inner image and a private, inner life. This is the territory of the phenomenological researcher. How successful such an enterprise is remains a matter of conjecture. The likelihood of a person – any person – opening themselves up to another person (in this case, the researcher) to such a degree that they are able to reveal the inner life, seems problematic. We should not claim too much for this approach, perhaps, and should be humble about the degree to which we ever can penetrate very far beneath the surface. If people are guarded and defensive about their inner lives, they are guarded and defensive for good reasons: this is what keeps them together for much of the time. Phenomenological research, then, should not be intrusive and is never a form of counselling or psychotherapy.

Philosophical background

Phenomenological research is linked to the branch of philosophy known as phenomenology, although those links should not be thought of as being as strong as they are sometimes held to be. It is easy to confuse a 'philosophy' with a 'research method', when the names are so similar. It should be remembered that philosophers are not normally researchers nor are they usually discussing theories about research, but more general theories about the world. It is still surprising to see philosopher's names invoked in the name of social sciences and health-care research, as if those philosophers had, at some point, contributed to healthcare research!

Phenomenology, as a philosophy, is concerned with the attempt to see things cleanly and 'as they really are'. When we look at things, in an everyday way, we label what we see in all sorts of ways. For example, we might say of a countryside scene: 'this is breathtaking: it is so beautiful!' In fact, in another sense, it is merely trees, grass and sky. We have overlaid the view with our own aesthetic value-judgements. Similarly, we may say about someone: 'he is such a kind, considerate man!' He may sometimes be these things and to some people. Equally, he may not always be these things and, to some people he may never be these things. What he is, in fact, is a mixture of physical properties with various psychological ones, some of which are more constant than others. What we have chosen to do when we describe him as 'kind and considerate' is to project on to him qualities that we appreciate and which we perceive him (possibly on little evidence) to have. Phenomenology, as a philosophy, aims at attempting to view things as they are stripped of such value judgements. The lofty aim of this enterprise is to get to 'the truth' but only acknowledging the brute fact of things. We must be careful, though, not to, too quickly, make the link between the philosophy and the research method.

Phenomenological research also has links with existential philosophy. Existentialists believe that we are the authors of our own lives. We are not born with a particular spirit, soul or predisposition. As soon as we become conscious enough to make decisions for ourselves, we begin to 'write ourselves': we begin to decide who we are. The reason we are able to do this, say the existentialists, is because we can exercise free will. Faced with a number of options, we are always able to choose what we do. The opposite of free will is determinism. This is the notion that the physical world around us is governed by deterministic principles. If we consider a household object such as a washing machine, before it was a washing machine, it was various pieces of metal and plastic. Before that metal and plastic existed, they were ore or coal tar. And so we can trace a direct, causal chain back through the history of the physical world around us. What makes human beings different, according to existential philosophers, is that people can choose and have consciousness. They can redirect their lives in a way that a washing machine cannot.

A third link with phenomenological research can be found in Buddhism. A major feature of Buddhist teaching is that all things, at all times, are changing. Nothing remains static. If this is true for the physical world, it is also true for the human world. Buddhists value, amongst other things, an acceptance of constant change and an attempt at perceiving the world *as it really is* – as opposed to overlaying what we see with all sorts of theoretical constructs and value judgements.

Thus, the recurrent themes that can be drawn from these philosophical roots are an acknowledgement that people invent their own lives and their own inner worlds; that it is interesting and instructive to attempt to see people as they really are and to view them in some depth; that, if we want to understand people, we must aim at viewing them with clear vision and not make attempts at interpreting what or who we think they are. Drawing from phenomenology as a philosophy, phenomenological researchers sometimes use the expression 'bracketing' to indicate the idea of attempting, as a researcher, to put aside your own thoughts, feelings and beliefs about a person and thus attempt to view them as they might view themselves. Perhaps this is similar to the psychotherapeutic concept of empathy, or the attempt at placing yourselves in the shoes of another person and viewing the world as they view it. The degree to which anyone can ever achieve any great degree of bracketing remains a contentious point.

Applications

So, how might all this apply to social science or healthcare research? For what might it be used and to what end? I can offer a personal example here. Over the last few decades, I have regularly been treated for depression. At times, I have pondered on what it is like for other people to be depressed. Do they feel the same as I do? Do they feel very, very different? What do they feel like when they are taking anti-depressants? What do they think about when they are depressed? In one sense, these questions could be answered with a simple 'symptoms checklist' and quantitative methods could be used to attempt to find out about the experience of depression. My view is that such methods would only amount to skating over the surface. Such methods would not produce the sort of data that would interest me. Phenomenological approaches to these questions could identify much deeper and more illuminating views of what it is like to be depressed. In turn, the answers to such questions could help in deciding how to help those who are depressed and could help in the education of those who care for the depressed. As we have seen before, the data obtained in this way would be 'illuminative'.

All this highlights, nicely, some of the important differences between quantitative and qualitative approaches to research. If we use the metaphor of a city, quantitative methods supply the important, numerical facts about the place. How many people live there? How much money is generated? And so on. Qualitative methods are like photographs of the place. They offer evidence of a different sort. Arguably, both forms of evidence are important. We need to know the facts and figures but we also need to know what a place looks like and how that view of it changes over time. Phenomenological research methods offer us snapshots of individual people's inner lives. Such views can aid in the understanding of what it is like to be variously human. We are not all the same – but neither are we all totally different. We can learn much from hearing, seeing and reading about other people's experiences. This is the basic material for phenomenological researchers.

Here are some more examples of questions where phenomenological research is useful.

Examples of phenomenological research questions

What is it like to experience major surgery?
How does it feel to experience loss?
What is the experience of having an MRI scan in the diagnosis of multiple sclerosis?
What is it like to spend long periods in hospital?
What does it feel like to be unable to walk for months on end, then to learn to walk again?

Again, all these questions could be answered structurally and, perhaps, superficially, with quantitative methods. Questionnaires could be devised which, in turn, produce the figures that identify parts of the answers to the questions. However, if we want to know more of the human side of the equation, we need to look more closely at individual human experience. Put simply, if you want to know about what someone thinks or feels – ask them.

Methods

Perhaps the most frequently used method of data collection, in phenomenological research, is the in-depth interview or series of interviews. Mostly, such interviews are relatively unstructured or open-ended. The interviewer may, for example, be very open and upfront about his aim and say to the respondent: 'I am interested in your experience of being depressed. I would appreciate anything you have to say on the issue...' Following this opening, the researcher might prompt the respondent, by using open questions or by asking for examples and elaborations. All the time, the researcher bears in mind that she is *not* attempting to compare and contrast this person's experience with that of others but attempting, instead, to capture this person's experience: as he or she tells it. The respondent, then, is telling a story and it is the researcher's task to help in the development and the elaboration of that story: not by adding to it, but simply by prompting and helping.

As with other qualitative approaches, it is usual to record phenomenological interviews. Mostly, this is done with the aid of a tape recorder or sometimes, by hand, in the form of detailed notes. The analysis of the data is not dissimilar to the content analysis described in Chapter 11. The researcher is careful, though, not to offer judgements and pseudo-explanations of what she thinks the respondent is talking about. The aim is to allow the respondent to describe their world view, with the researcher getting in the way as little as possible. Thus, the researcher, in her report, uses reported speech to illuminate the picture being painted by the respondent. She may also, from the interview data, offer an account of those respondents' theories about what is going on.

All of us carry with us a range of theories about how the world is. Sometimes these are informed, worked out and logical theories. Sometimes they are parts of our cultural folk law. Sometimes they are 'magical thinking': we simply hold odd views about things that go on in our heads and things that happen in the world. The phenomenological researcher is not interested in arguing with these, when she discovers them in the respondent, nor on offering a form of education to correct faulty beliefs. Instead, the researcher describes and continues to describe until she has created the clearest and most accurate picture of what the person in front of her 'is about'. This may be done by iteratively checking back with the respondent, as the research report is written. It is often useful for the researcher to go back and ask: 'is this what you meant? Or 'have I got this right?'

From the evidence-based healthcare point of view, phenomenological studies can offer vivid, personal insights into a range of issues to do with patient experience and care. By its nature, phenomenological reporting is always 'first person' and offers a direct account of what it feels like to be *this* person, in *this* situation, at *this* time. While we must exercise caution and resist a temptation to generalise from such studies, an interesting phenomenon is that which is sometimes called the 'phenomenological nod'. That is to say that when we read some subjective accounts of other people's lives, we find ourselves thinking: 'Yes! That is also true for me – but I hadn't thought of it in quite that way!' Phenomenological accounts can thus help us to reflect on our own practices as HCPs and, in this sense, can add, usefully, to the evidence bases of the professions.

Review questions

What is the main general aim of phenomenology?
How is it possible to see the world through someone else's eyes?
What does bracketing involve? How might this be accomplished?

Exercise

Can you really put yourself in the shoes of another person and see their world view? If someone were to try and do this with yourself, what would they find? Consider what thoughts, feelings and experiences make you the person you are? Now consider how someone else would go about finding these things out about you? Would interviewing be enough? How much interviewing? An hour? Several hours? A lifetime?

Further reading

Baker, J.D. (1997) Phenomenography: an alternative approach to researching the clinical decision making of nurses. *Nurse Inquiry*, 4(1), 41–47.

Beck, C.T. (1994) Phenomenology: its use in nursing research. *International Journal of Nursing Studies*, 31(6), 499–510.

Creswell, J.W. (2007) *Qualitative Inquiry and Research Design: Choosing Among Five Approaches*. London: Sage.

Langdridge, D. (2007) *Phenomenological Psychology: Theory, Research and Method*. London: Prentice Hall.

Mays, N. (ed.) (1995) *Qualitative Research in Health Care*. London: BMJ Books.

Moustakas, C.E. (1994) *Phenomenological Research Methods*. London: Sage.

Paley, J. (1998) Misinterpretive phenomenology: Heidegger, ontology and nursing research. *Journal of Advanced Nursing*, 27(4), 817–824.

A Pragmatic Approach to Qualitative Data Analysis

Introduction

Content analysis is used, as a phrase, in various ways. Mostly, though, it refers to the organising and ordering of textual data. Textual data can be of any sort – newspapers, books, interview transcripts, the 'grey

Research for Evidence-Based Practice in Healthcare, Second edition, by Robert Newell and Philip Burnard
© 2011 Robert Newell and Philip Burnard

literature' (literature that falls outside of that published in books and journals). All of this can be content analysed. Usually, though, it is a method used to analyse the text in transcriptions of interviews.

A transcription is the writing out of a recording of an interview. It is good practice to write down everything that is said. Sometimes the researcher herself does this transcribing. At other times, a clerk or copy typist is employed to do it. There is an argument that it is better for the researcher to transcribe his or her own interviews as this brings the research closer to the material that makes up the data. Another view is that typing transcripts is, largely, a clerical task that can be carried out by someone who is not a researcher. If this second option is available, however, the researcher must always check the typed transcript against the original tapes. It is quite possible for a typist to mishear a word or words being spoken. This is particularly the case when interviewees have broad or foreign accents. I (PB) recall conducting an ethnographic study about culture and communication in Thailand. Thai people, generally, speak quietly, and their accents, when speaking in English, are often fairly broad. As you will remember from Chapter 7, interviews for part of this study were also carried out in an environment that contained noisy air-conditioning equipment, and it soon became clear that tape recording of the interviews was not a reasonable option.

Although many researchers claim that tape recording interviews is almost essential in qualitative research, it became clear that taking notes, in this way, was a good second option. Very little appeared to be lost and it is surprising how much can be written down and how quickly. We intend to experiment with typing utterances directly into a small, notebook computer in further studies.

Content analysis can take a number of forms. Some of these will be discussed and then one method of undertaking the process will be described in more detail.

The most basic form of content analysis – and perhaps the one with most problems associated with it – is to obtain a computer program that records the number of times words are used in a transcript. Such a program lists, in descending order, the number of occurrences of words.

Word counts

The 1029
Beautiful 340
Artistic 239

Once such a listing has been obtained, it is then possible to exclude non-lexical words, such as 'the', 'to', 'that' and so on. What is left is an interesting array of the lexical words used in a transcript. Quite how useful such a listing is remains open to debate. If thought is given to how people talk, it will become evident that they may well repeat a given word many times. Consider, for example, this response to the question: 'what do you think about nursing models?'

> ### Example response
>
> 'Nursing models? Well, I think *some* nursing models...well, a few nursing models, anyway, can be quite useful. You know, if you are talking about nursing models and not nursing theories...now I am not sure what a nursing model is!'

In this example, the phrase 'nursing models' is used five times. It is not difficult to see that there may *not* be a relationship between how *often* a word appears in an interview and the *importance* of that word. We have used this method once and can offer an example of how the method can be used to highlight issues in a research project that were missed with other forms of analysis.

Some years ago, PB undertook a series of telephone interviews about the topic of HIV/AIDS counselling. Each of these was recorded and then a program was used to count the number of occurrences of lexical words in the transcripts. Other forms of data analysis were also used. What became clear was that the word 'anger' headed the list of lexical words, following this analysis. The author then returned to reading the transcripts and realised, for the first time, that the notion of anger *did* have a large part to play in the interviews. As I have noted, this was missed with other forms of data analysis.

Used with extreme caution, the word-count form of content analysis has its place in the analysis of textual data. However, care should be taken in making any detailed sort of *interpretation* of the data that arise out of this activity. The objective nature of the word count, can, most usefully, be combined with a more subjective review of the data in the light of this word-counting process. Word counting, alone, is not a useful or valid activity in qualitative research. If we were to draw an analogy with quantitative research, this kind of content analysis would be, at best, the equivalent of the simplest kinds of descriptive statistics, but possibly no more than frequency counts. In other words, this is merely presentation, rather than *transformation* of the data. In both quantitative and qualitative contexts, no meaning is either clarified or added at this simplest level.

Grounded theory

Although often written about as a research method in its own right, grounded theory is also an approach to analysing qualitative data. The idea behind grounded theory is that social facts 'emerge' out of the collected qualitative data, rather than the researcher being able, in some way, to 'divine' meanings about those data. An analogy that may help here is that of a block of marble prior to its being sculpted. The sculptor may argue that his projected horse is already 'in' the marble and it is his job to help it 'emerge'. Similarly, those who take a grounded theory approach to data may argue that meanings are already 'in' the data they collect and that it is their job to 'release' those meanings.

It is important to highlight the word 'theory' in this discussion. In the grounded theory literature, the aim is to use the emergent data to produce a theory which can then be further tested out. In our experience, quite a number of researchers who claim to do grounded theory seem to omit the theory. The whole point of grounded theory seems to be to collect rounds of data and to continue to refine the theory that emerges out of each round.

Grounded theorists, like ethnographers and those who use a phenomenological approach to research, still have to analyse their data into categories. There often appear to be great similarities in the ways that all qualitative researchers analyse their data. The rest of this chapter, then, is taken up with practical ways of analysing data and, we would argue, that can be used by those who do ethnographic, phenomenological or grounded theory approaches to research.

We appreciate that purists in each of these areas of qualitative research might argue that there are considerable differences in the ways they analyse data. If you are planning on doing a qualitative study, it is important to read widely around these topics.

Thematic content analysis

Frequently, in qualitative research, a form of 'thematic content analysis' is used to help organise and structure the data that accumulates from interviews. There are at least two opposing approaches to such analysis. The overall aim of both sorts of analysis is to first of all identify 'themes' or topics that occur in the data. Once these themes have been identified, the researcher can comb through the data for examples of utterances under each of these themes and cut and paste the data under these themed headings.

However, as noted above, there are at least two approaches to the identification of themes as part of such an analysis. The first might be called a 'template' approach. Here, the researcher asks questions of the dataset. Thus, in a series of interviews about health care education, the researcher might ask him or herself the questions: 'What did the interviewees say about teaching?', 'What did they say about evaluation?', 'What did they say about reflective practice?' and so on. In turn, each of the short versions of these questions becomes a *category*. Thus, in the example above, the first set of categories (or report sub-headings) are 'Teaching', 'Evaluation' and 'Reflective practice'.

The researcher continues to ask questions of the data, in this way, until he can account for almost everything that was said, by all the interviewees. Once this has happened, the data can be cut and pasted under the various headings generated in this way. A variant of this approach – particularly for a very large dataset – is for the researcher to pose *only* questions to which he is looking for an answer. Thus, his questions might be: 'What were the positive things said about teaching and learning methods?' and 'What were the negative things said about teaching and learning methods?' In this way, the researcher 'interrogates' the dataset and selects from it data about the particular and specific issues he is interested in and which will help to answer his research question.

The other approach to thematic content analysis is to adopt almost the opposite position to the data. In this method, the categories of data are said to 'emerge' from those data. It is the researcher's job, here, not to *look* for categories of information but to allow their *emergence*. What is more debatable, perhaps, is the degree to which categories ever do 'emerge' and to what degree the research 'looks' for them. As this is one of the most frequently used methods of content analysis of textual data, it will be described in more detail. The method described here is the one developed by one of us (PB) and which has been widely cited as a method of qualitative data analysis in other people's reports. The method, as described below, refers to the analysis of interview transcripts. However, it is quite possible to adapt the method for analysing any other form of texts (e.g. newspapers, handouts, curriculum documents, government reports).

A pragmatic approach to schematic content analysis

Stage one

Notes are made after each interview regarding the topics talked about during the interview. It is useful if the researcher writes herself 'memos' during the research project. A memo, in this case, is a short note about an idea, theory or any other mental activity that has taken place within the researcher. The idea of a 'memo' is similar to that of keeping field-notes – as we saw in Chapter 9. These memos serve as memory joggers and are useful, at a later date, when the researcher is writing up a report of his or her data.

Stage two

The interview transcripts are read through and notes made throughout the reading on general themes that appear in the transcripts. The aim, in general, is to become immersed in the data and to get to know it very well. Examples of general notes made, at this stage, might be as follows:

Early general notes in qualitative data analysis

- There seems to be a lot of discussion about student attitudes to teaching methods.
- Many respondents seem to worry about being understood!
- Some respondents are positive about reflective practice while others seem very against it ....

These notes can be written in the margins of the transcripts. Again, at a later date, they serve as memory joggers when the researcher comes to writing a report of the study.

Stage three

The researcher reads through the transcripts, again and again, and as many headings as necessary are written down to describe all aspects of the content. This stage is sometimes known as 'open coding': words and phrases are written in the margins of the transcripts that 'summarise' or categorise – what is being said by the respondents. An example of this form of coding is offered in Figure 11.1.

As can be seen, what happens in this stage is that the data are being categorised and that this, in turn, will lead to some *reduction* in text. Clearly, one option for the qualitative researcher would simply be to bind up all his or her interviews and to present them as his or her findings. Most people, however, would not consider this to be 'doing research'. Mostly, researchers are required to use as *much* of the qualitative data as possible, but it is also recognised that some of those data

Interview transcript	Examples of open coding
I think reflection can be important but it is not essential. A lot has been made of it in recent years and I think it might be over-rated. Many lecturers seem to like it but the students get bored when they are asked to keep those reflective journals. To be honest, I suspect some of them just make stuff up in them. I know I would!	Reflection is important Reflection not essential Reflection may be over-rated Students get bored with reflection Reflective journals Content of RJ made up?

Figure 11.1 Open coding of interview transcripts

must be lost. In the above example, for example, the researcher has ignored the comment, from the interviewee, that *he* would 'make things up' in a reflective diary. Clearly, these are subjective value judgements and the researcher has to think clearly about what he or she does or does not exclude.

Stage four

As the categories are collected together, it will be noticed that a number of them overlap. Consider, for example, the following (partial) list of category codes:

Initial category codes

- Reflection is important
- Reflective journals
- Teaching reflection
- The importance of reflection
- Dangers
- Anxiety about doing it right
- How to evaluate reflection?
- Educational issues
- Valuing reflection
- Worrying about reflection

First of all, the codes 'reflection is important' and 'valuing reflection' are so similar that one of the codes can be discarded. The next process is to see if other codes can be lumped together under higher order codes. In this way, the codes, themselves, are reduced. Consider, for example, how the above set of category codes might be subsumed under the following, shorter, set of codes.

Extended or 'collapsed' category codes

- **The value of reflection** ('Reflection is important', 'the importance of reflection', 'valuing reflection').
- **Reflection and educational issues** ('reflective journals', 'teaching reflection', 'how to evaluation reflection?', 'educational issues').
- **Personal reactions to reflection** ('anxiety about doing it right', 'dangers', 'worrying about reflection').

In this way, a smaller, more manageable set of category codes is developed. As a rule of thumb, it is better not to have more than about 12 final category codes in any given project. If the researcher generates more than this number, it is often difficult for him or her to keep in his or her mind the differences between them.

Stage five

The next stage is to return to the interview transcripts, armed with the shortened list of category codes. If the analysis is being done by hand (as opposed to being done with the help of a qualitative data management program such as *Atlas TI* or *The Ethnograph*), it is useful to have a set of brightly coloured, transparent ink, marker pens.

Each of these pens is allocated to a category code. In the above, short, set of categories for example, these may be as follows:

- **The Value of reflection**
- **Reflection and educational issues**
- **Personal reactions to reflection**

Next, the researcher works through the transcripts, marking up each part of the text, with the marker pens that reflect the category codes. Here is an example of that process.

Colour assignments to category codes

'I think reflection is very useful ... it helps me think about what I do in practice, as I go along. Before I just used to, like, do my work. Now I stop and think, every so often: "did I do that right? Could I have done it better?" My only real worry is I am not always sure if the lecturers in the college really know that much about it. Well, they know about the theory and can talk about that all day but I am not sure how many of them really know how to use it on the wards and things.'

Eventually, all the text in the transcripts is covered in the different colours of the marker pens that represent different category headings. Once this is done, the researcher draws vertical lines down the edge of each page of each interview. The first interview pages will have one vertical line in the margins, the second interview pages will have two vertical lines in the margins and so on. These are used to identify which passage of text came from which interview, once the pages are cut up.

After this, the researcher cuts up all the pages of interviews, according to the coloured sections. Then, all the pink sections are piled up together, all the lime green ones and so on. Finally, in this stage, all the pieces of text from a particular colour code can be stapled onto pages and filed together. The researcher ends up with a large file, divided with labelled index markers, containing (in each section) all the quotations under a particular heading.

To summarise: the text is marked up with marker pen. All the marked sections are cut up and filed, in separate sections of a large file, using index cards to separate each section. From experience, it is often best to use a lever arch file to contain this categorised data. Such a file can be opened completely flat – to allow access to the categorised data – and it can contain a fairly large dataset.

There is some controversy over whether or not the researcher should then return to some of his or her respondents and check the validity of his or her analysis. Those in favour of this approach suggest that checking back with respondents helps to add authority to the analysis: the respondents either do or do not agree with that analysis. Those against this approach suggest that this sort of checking is, in the end, impossible. The interviews from which the data came happened some time ago, the analysis has separated out sections of the interviews and no one can be expected to know whether or not the analysis is an 'accurate' one. From this perspective, the argument goes, the researcher should be prepared to stand by his or her own analysis: it is, after all, something of a subjective process.

Stage six

The organised data then forms the material from which the qualitative report is written. As we saw in Chapter 9, there are two options in writing up a qualitative findings section of a research report. The first option is to link the findings to previous research. The second option is to report only the findings and to make reference to other research only in a separate discussion section of the report. Here are three examples of the writing up of qualitative research findings, after the above analysis has taken place. Note that it is normally best to report such findings in a relatively 'flat' and descriptive way. This is not the time to speculate or theorise over what the findings may or may not 'mean'. If there is a place at all for this sort of activity, it is in a discussion section, after the presentation of findings. Some would argue that *all* that should be presented are the findings and that it is not the researcher's job to speculate and theorise – and certainly not to attempt to *generalise* from the findings. The third example, below, offers what might be deemed a 'bad' presentation of findings, in that the researcher has speculated well beyond his or her ability to do so, given the status of the data.

Write up of qualitative findings using references to other research

The value of reflection

A number of the respondents referred to how much they found reflection useful in their work as nurses. One suggested the following:

> *I use it everyday now. Once I got the hang of working out how to do it, I found myself thinking about what I do on the ward, when I got home in the evening. I sort of went through it, piece by piece, and wondered what were the best bits of what I did.*

This 'reflection after work' phenomenon is also noted in Green and Booker's (2004) study. In a survey of 403 third-year student nurses, Green and Booker found that 68% of their respondents described reflecting on practice after they had left the workplace.

Another, while finding reflection useful, questioned the time it took to use reflection – and particular reflection-in-action:

> *Yes, I think reflective practice is useful. It makes you think about what you do. I don't really understand how people can do that reflection-in-action thing, though. I work in a busy operating room and I just don't see how you can keep thinking about what you do, as you do it. That seems stupid to me.*

Black (2003), having undertaken a descriptive study of 315 clinical nurses, noted that many found difficult in both understanding the idea of reflection-in-practice and in being able to use it.

Write up of qualitative findings without reference to other research

The value of reflection

A number of the respondents referred to how much they found reflection useful in their work as nurses. One suggested the following:

> *I use it everyday now. Once I got the hang of working out how to do it, I found myself thinking about what I do on the ward, when I got home in the evening. I sort of went through it, piece by piece, and wondered what were the best bits of what I did.*

Another, while finding reflection useful, questioned the time it took to use reflection – and particular reflection-in-action:

> *Yes, I think reflective practice is useful. It makes you think about what you do. I don't really understand how people can do that reflection-in-action thing, though. I work in a busy operating room and I just don't see how you can keep thinking about what you do, as you do it. That seems stupid to me.*

Example of a poor write up of qualitative findings

The value of reflection

A number of the respondents referred to how much they found reflection useful in their work as nurses. One suggested the following:

> *I use it everyday now. Once I got the hang of working out how to do it, I found myself thinking about what I do on the ward, when I got home in the evening. I sort of went through it, piece by piece, and wondered what were the best bits of what I did.*

This 'reflection after work' phenomenon is also noted in Green and Booker's (2004) study. In a survey of 403 third-year student nurses, Green and Booker found that 68% of their respondents described reflecting on practice after they had left the workplace. Clearly, the respondent quoted above, showed how most nurses can benefit from using reflective practice. While it continues to grow in popularity, it is important that more and more colleges of nursing use it in their curricula to promote good practice.

Another respondent, while finding reflection useful, questioned the time it took to use reflection – and particular reflection-in-action:

> *Yes, I think reflective practice is useful. It makes you think about what you do. I don't really understand how people can do that reflection-in-action thing, though. I work in a busy operating room and I just don't see how you can keep thinking about what you do, as you do it. That seems stupid to me.*

This respondent clearly does not understand the notion of reflection-in-practice. She makes the common mistake of dismissing the concept on the basis of her own misunderstanding of it. It seems likely that the quality of teaching about reflective practice, in her college of nursing, was very poor. More time needs to be set aside in colleges to make sure that all students are thoroughly aware of what is to be gained by using reflection-in-practice.

In this final example, whilst the researcher has adopted the 'discussion with findings' approach, the account lacks transparency, because the researcher has also intruded into the account with unsubstantiated value judgements of her own. Sometimes, in poor quality reports of qualitative data analysis, the distinction between findings, references to other literature and authorial comment is so blurred as to be entirely opaque to reader and to prevent the respondent's voice from emerging.

Conclusion

This chapter has identified one approach to the analysis of qualitative data. While the examples are from (imaginary) interview transcripts, the method described here could easily be adapted to suit other media, such as text from magazines and books, notebooks containing a researcher's field notes and so on. In the end, what the method is describing is a means of handling and organising *text*. And, arguably, text – in all its varieties – is the basic material in almost all qualitative research projects.

Review questions

Is content analysis itself a method of data analysis at all?
What are the two approaches to thematic content analysis described here?
What are the six stages in the pragmatic approach to thematic content analysis?

Exercise

If you have already reached the data analysis stage of a project of your own, why not use the pragmatic approach to analysis described here to analyse it? If not, a page of newspaper text offers an easy possibility to practice data analysis.

Further reading

Boeije, H.R. (2009) *Analysis in Qualitative Research*. London: Sage.

Burnard, P. (1991) A method of analysing interview transcripts in qualitative research. *Nurse Education Today*, 11, 461–466.

Meho, L.I. (2006) E-mail interviewing in qualitative research: a methodological discussion. *Journal of the American Society for Information Science and Technology*, 57(10), 1284–1295.

Silverman, D. (1997) *Qualitative Research: Theory, Method and Practice*. London: Sage.

Wainwright, S.P. (1994) Analysing data using grounded theory. *Nurse Researcher*, 1(3), 43–49.

Wise, C., Plowfield, L.A., Kah, D.L. and Steeves, R.H. (1992) Using a grid for interpretation and presenting qualitative data. *Western Journal of Nursing Research*, 14(6), 796–800.

Website

http://hsc.uwe.ac.uk/dataanalysis/qualWhat.asp

Limitations of Qualitative Research

Key points

- Qualitative research does not claim to be scientific in the same way as quantitative research.
- Samples in qualitative research are rarely representative.
- The researcher's own influence on the emerging data may be checked by bracketing and by discussion with respondents.
- There is too much variability to allow replication of qualitative studies.
- Qualitative research does not aim to generalise.
- Neither researcher nor respondent is necessarily aware of their own biases.
- Analysis of interviews can be affected by hindsight bias.
- Validation by respondents is itself potentially problematic.
- Respondents can offer explanations about things they have no way of knowing about.
- The illuminative value of quantitative research is slowly gaining ground in healthcare.

Research for Evidence-Based Practice in Healthcare, Second edition, by Robert Newell and Philip Burnard
© 2011 Robert Newell and Philip Burnard

Introduction

Qualitative research methods are valuable in helping to gather descriptions of other people's ideas, thoughts, feelings, attitudes and values. As we have noted, the most commonly used data collection method is the interview, while the most frequently used method of data analysis is a version of content analysis.

Qualitative approaches to healthcare research are of a more recent origin than quantitative. Also, such approaches do not, necessarily, follow the scientific method seen in quantitative research. The degree to which the scientific approach can be applied to human beings, given their difference to other objects in the world is a matter of debate. The fact that people have consciousness and can think and ponder on their situation, means that quantitative data may not best represent a given person's situation over time. Put simply, we can change our minds. This, in turn, means that *any* form of research into human subjects can only ever offer a glimpse of a situation at a particular time and in a particular context. We would, then, be advised to be careful about the degree to which we generalise our findings in any human research.

In this chapter, the limitations of the qualitative approach to research are examined. It should be noted, in advance, that – perhaps because of its newness and difference from quantitative research – some of those in the health and caring professions still view it with suspicion. Some also compare the approach rather too directly with quantitative research and expect the rules of quantitative research to apply to qualitative. They do not. We are both members of Local Research Ethics Committees. Such committees are in place throughout the UK to consider and approve medical and healthcare proposals. Any research that is likely to involve patients or healthcare workers has, first, to be approved by such committees. We are still surprised by the questions sometimes raised about qualitative proposals (e.g. 'Where is the hypothesis?', 'Isn't this study a rather subjective one?'). To raise these questions, as we have noted in previous chapters, is to miss the point of qualitative research. The point in, such work, is to describe and to collect subjective views from a range of people. Qualitative research findings cannot, by the nature of the sampling and data collection methods used, be generalised out to larger populations. The point of qualitative research is to describe and illuminate.

It would be a mistake, then, to criticise qualitative research in terms of the conditions applied to quantitative. The enterprise does not claim to be a 'scientific' one in the commonly accepted sense. Indeed, many qualitative commentators would question the degree to which *any* human research can be scientific. However, we cannot reject all the criticisms laid against qualitative research and it will be valuable to explore some of them.

Reliability and validity

These general concepts are examined in Chapter 6. Put simply, qualitative and quantitative researchers are generally united in the view that the entity being examined (rather than something else) should emerge from the results of a study (validity) and that it should do so in a systematised way (reliability). However, in qualitative research, those issues are not so clear-cut as they are in quantitative. There are, perhaps, three reasons for this.

First, the sampling methods used in qualitative research are rarely, if ever, representative. No attempts are made to obtain random samples from a larger population. Instead, as we have seen, samples are usually *convenience* or *purposive* and sometimes both. A convenience sample is one that 'is to hand': it is made up of people who are prepared to take part in the study. A purposive sample is a sample of people who are likely to have a view on the topic that is being investigated. Given that sampling is not randomised and, therefore, not representative of a larger population, we cannot fully address sampling validity issues in qualitative research.

Second, data collection methods, in qualitative studies, usually involve either semi-structured interviews or observation. Both of these methods have built-in problems in terms of keeping everything uniform. One interview may not be anything like the others, in a series. Interviews may vary in terms of their overall 'quality', their tone, and so on, over time. Again, these are a threat to both the validity and reliability of the project.

Third, people, themselves, are variable. As we shall see, people may give different responses to different people, they may offer different views on different days. Similarly, the researchers' own 'changeability' comes into the equation: one researcher's treatment of a qualitative dataset may be quite different from that of a colleague. In quantitative research (as long as the appropriate procedures are followed) this variability is not the case: a range of quantitative researchers, handling the same dataset, with the same computer program, will come up with the same results. The findings in a qualitative study are not so likely to be so 'clean' in this way and this further limits the degree to which we can claim to have carried out a reliable and valid study.

However, we can, as far as possible, undertake certain checks in these respects. By attempting to 'bracket' or put to one side our own views on the topic being researched, we can cut down the likelihood of our bringing our own views into the analysis and subsequent discussion of data and findings. We can also check our analysis of the data with another research to see whether or not there is a reasonable case for our being able to say that we have been as objective and careful in our analysis as is possible. This checking process is not without its own problems. We might want to say that simply asking another colleague to check our system of analysis is to, potentially, bring in another level of error. With a check of this sort, we may also pick up the second researcher's biases.

Another device that is sometimes used for checking the appropriateness and validity of our analysis of the data is to discuss that analysis with the respondents, after the event. Again, such a system is hardly flawless. It seems likely that the respondents will not, themselves, be researchers and may have no comments to make on the processes that were completed. The respondents may also be pleasantly or unpleasantly surprised by the analysis and suggest changes based on this. Finally, the respondents may simply accept what the researcher has done – believing, perhaps, that the 'researcher knows best'.

In a well designed, quantitative study, an important feature is that a study should be able to be replicated and similar findings be found (once it is established that the original study's processes were sound). In qualitative research, it is rare that this is the case – and mostly for the reasons identified above. There are too many uncontrolled variables and possible sources of error for qualitative studies to be able to be replicated and similar findings identified. This is not so much of a limitation of the qualitative approach, but more an appreciation that the qualitative process is a very different one to the quantitative.

Many of the points in this section are revisited in the sections that follow. It is the *subjective* nature of qualitative research that is so often a problem for those who would question the usefulness of it. It is a subjective process both from the points of view of the respondents and also from the point of view of the researcher. It will be useful, therefore, to revisit some of the above points in a slightly different context.

Two overriding points need to be made in respect of a general approach to validity and reliability. First, the qualitative researcher must, like all researchers, be as honest and as careful in her work on any given project. Second, the researcher should always look for *disconfirmation* of her findings. At all stages, through the analysis and writing up of a qualitative project, the researcher should be asking: 'have I got this right?', 'is something else going on here?' or 'could things be otherwise?' Most research yields up new knowledge in very small increments. Any researcher – including the qualitative researcher – should be wary of any findings that seem very different from what has gone before. All researchers should, by nature perhaps, be conservative and not prone to expect large numbers of new findings. If such findings *are* forthcoming, they should ring a bell of caution in the head of the researcher. Such unusual new findings often, in the end, point to errors in the research process or to faulty assumptions on the part of the researcher.

Generalisability

Bearing in mind the point, made above, that the aim of qualitative research is not to generalise, it still remains a limitation of the approach. If research is intended to inform practice, then we might hope that we can draw evidence from it to apply to situations other than the ones dealt with in the research. Qualitative research is very limited in this respect. We cannot take a group of people's views and apply them to another context, another place or another group of people. We may read them and think 'Yes! This sounds familiar to me!' or 'I am surprised at these findings!' but we cannot, then, extrapolate from them and decide that we have hard evidence that can be applied in other contexts.

It is interesting to read the conclusions drawn from many qualitative studies. Some contain recommendations. These are sometimes in the format seen in quantitative studies, where the researcher suggests changes or modifications to practice that might result from considering the findings. It is arguable, given the points noted above, that qualitative researchers *cannot* make such recommendations. If it is true that findings from such studies are limited to a particular time, place and sample, then it follows that such findings should not generate recommendations for other times, places and populations.

Such lack of generalisability does not, however, mean that qualitative findings are not of value. As we have noted, qualitative work illuminates, offers glimpses of how other people work and think. Such findings can help us consider our own situation and learn from the thoughts, feelings and actions of others. They can allow us to compare and contrast our own views of practice with those of others. The limitation does mean, though, that we must always bear this 'generalisation' rule in mind and not automatically conclude that we have obtained hard evidence to apply to our own practice. This tendency to offer recommendations and advice to others at the end of qualitative research reports is often to be noted in those who are new to qualitative methods (although it is a tendency not always missing in those with considerable experience, either!).

The nature of human beings

Human beings, because of the fact of their consciousness, are in a constant state of flux and change. If we pause, for a moment, and consider our own thinking processes, we may note that such processes are not linear: we do not, necessarily, think logically or consistently. We are affected by our emotions, by the situation we find ourselves in and – sometimes – simply by whim. We are often contradictory in the things we think. A simple, everyday example, may serve to illustrate this. If we are driving a car and another driver forces his way in front of us, we consider this bad driving. If, however, we force our own way through traffic, we may feel that what we do is necessary. We often have one rule for ourselves and another for other people.

Similarly, we can very easily change our minds and our views. What I believed two years ago, I may not believe today: what I thought to be the case, yesterday, may not be what I believe today. This must be an important challenge for the qualitative researcher, who, it would seem, is committed to capturing the thoughts, feelings and actions of others. What such researchers may have caught is merely a snapshot of a person's thoughts, on a given day, in a particular situation. If the researcher were to conduct interviews with this person, on a different day or in a different context, he or she might gather very different data. The question must therefore be asked: 'To what degree are these findings, to any degree, an accurate representation of what another person thinks or feels?'

We also react to different people in different ways. When we are interviewed, we are also reacting to the person conducting the interview. Do we like him or her? Do we feel intimidated, threatened, superior or inferior to him or her? What, do we consider, is his or her motives in asking a question? What will he or she do with our utterances? These factors and many more influence the sort of responses we make to the questions we are asked. Most people, as students, have experienced the situation, in a classroom or lecture theatre, in which, on being asked a question by a lecturer, have thought: 'What *sort* of answer is required here?' Similarly, in research interviewing, the subject attempts to best-guess the response that they believe is being asked for. We do not simply offer an honest and open response. We modify our replies in accordance with all sorts of feelings and views we have about what is going on at the time.

Perhaps the most clear-cut example of this takes place in a job interview. Our responses to questions are clearly aimed at 'making a good impression'. We are, for obvious reasons, trying to present ourselves in the best possible light. We may exaggerate our good points and play down our weaker ones. Issues of confidence, self esteem and self-concept also come into play in the research interview. Few of us, in any situation, want to present ourselves in a bad light. We want other people to like us and we want to be appreciated. We may even want to offer what we perceive to be the 'right' answer.

An example, from a cultural study, conducted by one of the writers may help to illustrate this. The study was conducted in Thailand, where one of the cultural norms is to be polite and not to argue or contradict those perceived as being in a superior or 'one-up' position. The researcher visited a restaurant, in Thailand, with a respondent in the study. He noted that the owner of the restaurant was Chinese and (for reasons not, now clear) pointed this out to the respondent, who agreed.

The researcher and respondent met on other occasions and the restaurant became known, by shorthand, as the Chinese restaurant (even though it only served Thai food). In a later exchange, the researcher pondered on where, in China, the owner might have come from. The respondent replied that the owner had probably never been to China, as that owner was Thai!

The example illustrates a complicated, cultural issue. First, the researcher offered a flat, unquestioned, view of the origins of the owner. In order for the researcher not to 'lose face' the respondent did not challenge or deny the assertion. Only later, and possibly with some difficulty, did the respondent point out the mistake that had been made. If further exchanges had not taken place, the mistake may have remained unchallenged.

In this case, the researcher quickly learned not to make such flat assertions and, working with a Thai co-researcher, often checked assumptions and ideas about 'what was going on' to clarify and modify his understanding. However, it seems fairly likely that, in many qualitative studies, (a) assumptions are made and go unchallenged and (b) respondents, for various reasons, attempt to 'keep the researcher happy'.

All of this is complicated by the fact that we often do not appreciate our own biases and prejudices: we simply cannot account for all the things that we think and believe. This is true for both researcher and respondent. The researcher is often blind to his or her own values and beliefs and so is the respondent. Thus, the reporting, by both parties, of a clean and accurate account of any given situation seems fraught with difficulty. Errors, of varying degrees can creep into a study both from researchers and respondents. If the findings from such studies are then built into a 'theory' or into 'recommendations', errors may be built upon errors.

If it is true that respondents are changeable and that their thought processes vary from day to day, it is also true for researchers. The researcher may well analyse data some time after they are collected. This allows time for further errors to emerge. The research has to attempt to recall the interview and reconstruct it in his or her mind. However, many life events have taken place since the original encounter and it seems unlikely that recall of the interview, after the event, is necessarily an accurate one. The views of conversations emerging from a tape recorder or from written notes are not going to be the same as the ones that took place in real-time.

Data analysis

We have already noted one problem of data analysis. Analysis cannot, normally, take place as interviews happen (although the researcher is probably making some initial attempt at analysis during an interview).

The most detailed analysis takes place after the event. As we have noted, this can lead to bias. Our memory of events is rarely accurate – even if we have recorded interviews carefully. Our 'reading' of an interview, at a later date, is likely to be different to the reading of it as it took place. The 'live' interview is quite different to the recorded one.

One of us recalls, in a different study, undertaking a fairly lengthy interview and being impressed by the quality of that interview. He felt that much ground had been covered and that many useful things had been gleaned from the encounter. He was surprised, some time later, on playing back the tape of the interview that he found it very difficult to understand what had taken place! The 'good' interview had become difficult to fathom. Live interviews involve a range of dynamics that simply cannot be captured on tape or in notes. In a live interview, we respond to each other, we smile, use eye contact and understand each other in ways that are not easily recorded. Perhaps, in the future, more use will be made of visual as well as audio recording – both as means of data collection and as means of data reporting. However, it seems unlikely that any sort of recording will ever quite capture the atmosphere and the shared meanings that are present in the original encounter.

In most forms of the content analysis of qualitative data, the processes are subjective ones. Although, in the *grounded theory* approach to qualitative research, it is often claimed that data categories 'emerge' out of the data, it seems obvious to both of us that it is the *researcher* who devises those categories. To argue that such categories emerge is similar to saying that a block of stone 'contains' the eventual sculpture that the skilled artist produces. There is no sculpture in the block of stone until the sculptor fashions it. Similarly, there are no categories in a series of interview transcripts until the researcher develops them. And that process cannot be seen as an objective process. In the end, the qualitative researcher has to decide upon a series of headings – of his or her devising – and then identify which elements of the data fit under those headings. We might argue, then, that a different researcher might devise a different set of headings or that he or she might file data under those headings in quite a different way. These facts also point to another form of potential limitation: we cannot guarantee the relationship between the original dataset and what the researcher does with that dataset.

In summary then, we might say that, on a different day, with a different researcher, the data produced in a qualitative study may be different from *this* particular set. We might further say that what the researcher does when he or she analyses those data may vary from what another researcher might do. In the end, we are left to note a certain *arbitrariness* in the qualitative research process. We cannot argue that what we have captured, in any given study, is a clear picture of a person or persons' views, nor that the findings we have can, in any sense, be extrapolated out to other groups of people. We are left, in the most extreme view, with a very particular interpretation of a very particular situation.

We might elaborate this just a little further. It seems possible that a respondent, reading what has been done with the data he or she has supplied might have a variety of responses to the account. He or she might say, at least:

(a) Yes! I agree with this account! It is a very fair representation of what I said and what I believe to be true.

(b) Yes! I agree that this is what I said at the time... however, on re-flection, I was wrong and I no longer feel that this represents what I believe to be true.

(c) No! This is not an accurate representation of what I said.

Oddly enough, although the first option seems the most reassuring one, we might even question the holding of this view. If we believe, as seems to be borne out by our everyday experience, that people are dynamic, changing beings, we might wonder at a person's ability to make such a statement with any conviction! The second option is likely to trouble us, perhaps, and make us wonder about the validity of what we have done as researchers and to question, in various ways, the value of doing a qualitative study. The third option, perhaps, might lead us to believe we have done 'bad research' and not been careful enough in our procedures. However, as we have noted, perhaps we should not be surprised if the third option came to be expressed, occasionally, given the seeming arbitrariness of the processes involved in analysing qualitative data.

Despite all this, we can, I believe, justify the use of qualitative methods in an almost *literary* way. We can, perhaps, view qualitative data as a series of *stories*. A moment's thought will reveal that many aspects of our lives involve what might be called 'storytelling'. First, we tell ourselves stories. We invent reasons for why we and others do things. We offer ourselves explanations for our own and other people's behaviours, thoughts and feelings. We also offer other people stories. An example might be as follows. One of us, when driving into the centre of Cardiff, a busy capital city, will often comment, to his wife, on how it is busy on that day. On almost every occasion, his wife offers an 'explanation' of why that is the case (e.g. 'People are getting out earlier to the shops, today' or 'People want to get to be able to park in town'). These are examples of 'stories': the author's wife clearly cannot *know* why the city seems busy nor even know if the city is any busier than usual! In this way, though, we tell each other stories.

Similarly, in qualitative research, we are, perhaps, presented with stories about human lives, groups and cultures. Such stories should not be read too literally – for the reasons, at least, discussed above. Those stories can, however, help us to appreciate, a little more clearly, some aspects of the human condition. They illustrate human lives in a way that statistical information cannot. We can read these stories and, again, have various reactions to them, for example:

(a) Yes! I can understand this person's point of view and his or her experiences.
(b) What this person says surprises me.
(c) I do not believe what I am reading.
(d) I had never thought about this before, in this sort of way.

Clearly, many other reactions are possible, but the point is that the stories that emerge out of qualitative data are not necessarily versions of 'the truth' (and, in the end *no* research is offering that). Instead, they are illuminative accounts that help us to think more clearly – or in different ways – about a healthcare topic. Or they allow us glimpses of aspects of the human condition of which, before, we were unaware. For these reasons, perhaps, qualitative research – although of a different type and order to quantitative – can be found to be valuable.

From the point of view of evidence-based healthcare, qualitative methods are taking their time in being accepted as mainstream. One reason for this is the problem of generalisation: while it is possible to generalise from quantitative studies, such generalisation is not possible from qualitative studies. However, hopefully, the *illuminative* aspect of qualitative research will soon be more widely recognised and appreciated. We need human, subjective accounts of life (and death) alongside the more objective, detached, quantitative ones. Quantitative research cannot account for all aspects of the human condition – particularly for the more personal, subjective aspects. To some degree, these *can* be captured in qualitative research, and qualitative accounts can be very useful in attempting to offer the evidence base a personal view of healthcare. Or, to put it another way: where people are concerned, you cannot simply *count* everything.

Review questions

What are the main obstacles to generalising from qualitative research?

If qualitative research is limited by lack of generalisability, in what ways can it inform our practice?

Exercise

What stories did you tell yourself today? Think back and recall a couple of examples of plausible explanations you thought of for the behaviours of others or for your own behaviour. What 'real' evidence did you have for any of these explanations?

Further reading

Avis, M. and Robinson, J. (1996) Continuing dilemma in health care research. *NT Research*, 1(1), 9–11.

Baum, F. (1995) Researching public health: behind the qualitative–quantitative methodological debate. *Social Science and Medicine*, 40(4), 459–468.

Bryman, A. (1992) *Quantity and Quality in Social Research*. London: Routledge.

Newman, I. and Benz, C.R. (1998) *Qualitative–Quantitative Research Methodology: Exploring the Interactive*. Carbondale: Southern Illinois University Press.

SECTION 3
Quantitative Approaches

Sampling, Reliability and Validity Issues in Data Collection and Analysis

Key points

- Random sampling decreases the likelihood that members of a sample are different from its population.
- Stratification and cluster sampling both ensure adequate representation of population subgroups in a sample.
- Quota sampling and systematic sampling approximate to random sampling.
- Convenience sampling is the simplest form of sampling but is least likely to conform to its population.
- External validity refers to the applicability of a study to the real world.
- Population validity refers to the similarity between a study sample and its population.
- Ecological validity refers to the similarity between study conditions and procedures and the real world.
- Internal validity determines the confidence we can have in cause–effect relationships in a study.
- Reliability consists of two concepts: consistency and repeatability.

Research for Evidence-Based Practice in Healthcare, Second edition, by Robert Newell and Philip Burnard
© 2011 Robert Newell and Philip Burnard

> - Consistency implies that, if a phenomenon is unchanged, it will be measured as the same by several observers or by several measuring methods.
> - Repeatability means that, if a phenomenon is unchanged, it will be measured as the same on several occasions.

Introduction

In Chapter 6, we noted how, in sampling, quantitative researchers were concerned with the notion of representativeness and how this might be established by adequacy of sampling. This chapter explores some of the techniques used principally by quantitative researchers to increase the likelihood that their sampling approaches will lead to generalisable results. Other major issues which contribute to generalisability of a study are the reliability and validity of the ways in which data have been collected. We will introduce these later in this chapter, and they will be returned to in later chapters in the contexts of the types of research design they relate to.

Representativeness, fairness and random sampling

One important issue in establishing representativeness is the notion that each potential participant has a fair, equal chance of participating in a study. This is achieved principally by random sampling, which we touched on in Chapter 6. The most efficient way of creating a random sample is by the use of a computer-generated list of random numbers. Other methods such as putting numbers into a hat or tossing a coin are generally subject to human error or depart from true randomness for other reasons such as the fact that a small number of trials is rarely random.

Coin-toss experiment

Try tossing a coin 10 times, now.
Did you get 5 heads and 5 tails?
If so (possible but unlikely), try again?
Another 5 heads and 5 tails? We do not think so.
If you *did not* get 5 heads and 5 tails (likely), you probably do not think there is anything wrong with the coin – it is not heavier on one side, for example. This is because we all know, from our ordinary lives, that probabilities of this type take a long time to

even out. The same thing applies in research situations, too. Yet, randomisation by coin-toss was for many years to be thought to be adequate.

In surveys of a defined population, the researcher uses computer-generated numbers to choose which members of that population to enter into the study as the eventual sample, whilst in randomised controlled trials (see Chapter 17), a broadly similar process is used to assign participants to one treatment rather than another. Again, the notion of fairness is at the root of the procedure. The researcher is concerned that all participants have a fair chance of being allocated to each of the possible treatments. In the first instance, representativeness is increased because random selection reduces the likelihood that members of the sample are different from the whole population. In the second, it is increased because randomness decreases the likelihood that participants in one treatment are different from those in the other(s). In this second case, we are able to generalise from the sample to the supposed population because we assume that results in a population if they were similarly randomised would be equivalent to those in the sample. As we shall see in Chapters 15, 16 and 17, there are numerous other issues which affect our ability to make such a generalisation with confidence, but adequate randomisation is a basic prerequisite for drawing conclusions about populations from samples.

Stratification

In random sampling, stratification is one way of increasing fairness and, by extension, representativeness. At first glance, it might seem that, having sampled randomly, no further effort is required to ensure either of these things. For extremely large samples, this may, indeed, be true. However, most studies, even those with considerable samples, are not actually large enough to ensure fairness of inclusion. This is because, in many instances, populations are heterogeneous and practically sized samples are not large enough to capture that diversity. An extreme example will make this obvious. Breast cancer is extremely rare in males (roughly 1% of new UK cases annually). To be representative, we should ideally wish to sample 1 male patient for every 99 females. If we randomly sampled breast cancer patients, it is very unlikely that we would achieve this because the smaller the probability of something occurring in a given population, the larger the sample needed to capture it. In stratification, this problem is overcome by identifying sample numbers *in proportion* to the existence of different subgroups in the total population, then sampling at the same rate from each of the strata. In our example, we would identify say 100 men and 9900 women, and sample at a rate of 10% from each. We would then end up with an eventual sample of 10 men and 990 women, accurately reflecting the population of breast cancer patients. This is obviously a very large sample, but still much smaller that we would require to represent the genders fairly through randomisation alone. Characteristics such as gender, age and ethnicity are routinely stratified for in large studies, and stratification can also be applied to the allocation of patients to treatments in comparison studies such as RCTs.

Cluster sampling

This method of sampling is very close to stratification in that it is a way of ensuring fair representation of particular groups. It is done by randomly choosing particular *clusters* of participants. These clusters are typically geographical areas, but could, for example, also be hospital wards or diagnostic groups. It usually works most fairly if some form of comparability between the clusters can be reasonably asserted. Participants are then randomly chosen from within each cluster, typically, in accordance with the comparative size of the clusters. Cluster sampling is sometimes referred to as multistage sampling because of this second random sampling procedure. It would be possible to further break down each cluster into sub-clusters before eventually assigning participants.

The essential difference between stratified sampling and cluster sampling is that in cluster sampling, the clusters are chosen randomly from a larger population of clusters. In stratified sampling, *all* theoretically possible clusters are included and sampled from.

Cluster randomisation is a variant of cluster sampling used in treatment comparison studies (typically, RCTs), in which a treatment is randomly assigned to a setting. All patients who are treated in that setting who enter the study receive that treatment.

In high-quality quantitative research, the above methods of sampling are the most common, and are referred to as methods of *probability sampling*, because the probability of a participant appearing in a sample is equal to their rates in the population from which that sample is drawn. There are, however, numerous methods of *non-probability* sampling. Some of these are particularly associated with qualitative research, and are described in Chapter 7. Others are used in both quantitative and qualitative research. In quantitative research, they are regarded as less robust than probability samples, because their generalisability is poorer, and quantitative research typically has the aim of drawing inferences about populations from samples.

Quota samples

Quota sampling is perhaps closest to a probability sample, in that considerable efforts may be made to ensure representativeness. Researchers decide on a range of sampling parameters (*quota controls*) which are relevant to their study (e.g. age, gender, qualification, ethnic background) and sample on the basis of these. The difference between quota sampling and stratified sampling is that the numbers in each quota eventually recruited as participants via quota sampling do not necessarily reflect the rates of people in the study population who possess the quota control characteristics (although they may do). Even where the quotas do contain numbers of participants reflective of base levels, they are not selected randomly. Confusingly, some books refer to quota sampling as a type of stratified sampling (or the reverse). We prefer to use the term *stratification* only for random samples, as we believe this avoids confusion.

Systematic samples

Systematic sampling once again attempts to introduce fairness into the selection process. It involves the use of fixed intervals in assigning participants to a study. Thus, every fifth person from a list might be included in the sample. It is sometimes suggested that, if the first person to be drawn from the list is selected at random, before starting to pick every fifth person, then systematic sampling is a method of probability sampling. However, there is a possibility of biased sampling in systematic sampling. In the event that some bias has entered into compiling the list from which participants are to be drawn, then random assignment of the first participant will not help with this. It simply means that the biased list starts in a random place. This weakness is not present in random sampling, and therefore, whilst acknowledged to be a reasonably robust way of assigning participants to a study, systematic sampling is likely always to be less robust than random sampling, particularly where a list contains particular order characteristics the researcher is not aware of.

Convenience/accidental samples

This is probably the weakest form of sampling. It is also the easiest to obtain, and therefore the one most often seen in small projects and student assignments. The amount of generalisability possible from such a sample is low because of the inherent weaknesses in the sampling procedure. Convenience samples (sometimes called accidental samples) are exactly what they say, samples of people gained in the way most convenient to the researcher. This may be as simple as sampling patients by taking the next 100 who walk through the clinic door and asking them to complete a questionnaire, or taking the books at my bedside as a sample of my reading habits. However, supposing we take our sample of patients on a Monday, and the clinic always sees its sickest patients on that day. Similarly, supposing I like to read undemanding detective stories at night because they help me sleep, but have bookcases stacked with plays, non-fiction works etc., which I read extensively at other times. In both these extreme cases, the poor generalisability of convenience samples is evident. The same principle (that circumstances may introduce bias into convenience sampling) is just as problematic in all convenience sampling. Balanced against this shortcoming, convenience samples are the easiest to obtain, and this may be a critical factor in student projects or small pilot studies.

> **Synopsis of sampling approaches in quantitative research**
>
> Random sampling is most likely to ensure that a sample is generally representative of its population.
> In practice, stratification and cluster sampling refine random sampling in small samples to ensure adequate representation of subgroups.
> Non-random quota sampling and systematic sampling approximate to random sampling in their representativeness.
> Convenience sampling is weak because there is less likelihood of similarity between sample and population.

Sampling, representativeness and external validity

In Chapter 6, we encountered the notion of external validity (basically the applicability of study findings to the world at large), and how this was associated with the idea of representativeness. Adequate sampling is a key way of ensuring external validity, with the random sample achieving the highest level of such validity, and convenience sampling the lowest. A high degree of similarity between a study sample and its population is said to result in high *population* validity. The other way of increasing external validity is to ensure that the circumstances in which a study is conducted adequately reflect circumstances in the real world. This match between the study situation and the world is referred to as *ecological* validity, and issues surrounding it are discussed further in our discussion of external validity in Chapter 17.

Internal validity

Internal validity is essential to the establishment of cause–effect relationships and refers to the strength of relationships between different elements of a study. The notion of cause–effect relationships and how to establish them is described further in Chapters 14, 15 and 17, but an understanding of internal validity is basic to these discussions. In particular, the great majority of the discussion of the control of bias in these chapters is essentially a discussion of how to increase internal validity and, therefore, our confidence that the assumed cause–effect relationships we see are in fact the result of interactions between what we assume to be the cause and its assumed effects, rather than something else we have not considered. Polgar and Thomas (1997) identify three elements of internal validity: cause must precede effect; size of effect varies with size of cause; rival potential causes can be ruled out. The more these three conditions are satisfied, the greater the internal validity of the study.

For example, in a study of physiotherapy intervention with fatigue, we would be more confident that the action of the physiotherapist was responsible for reduction in patient fatigue if (a) reduction in fatigue only (or mostly) occurred after the intervention, (b) the greater the amount of intervention, the greater the reduction in fatigue and (c) the patient was having no other treatments or life changes which could account for the reduction in fatigue.

Reliability

Reliability consists of two concepts: consistency and repeatability. These ideas are usually associated with measurement, and we will deal with it in this context in the next section. However, as with many concepts in research, reliability is used in an everyday sense, too, and also contains the ideas of repeatability and consistency when used in this everyday sense. So, for example, when we speak of a reliable friend, we implicitly embrace the idea that we can trust that person to be roughly the same in different situations which demand similar responses (say, her sympathy or help), and roughly the same in those responses over time (at least in the short to medium term). Here, we are describing consistency and repeatability, respectively. Similarly, in healthcare, when we speak of improving the reliability of healthcare delivery, we are talking essentially about decreasing unwanted variation – ensuring that services are delivered consistently and repeatably across the country. Finally, in research, reliability carries these two meanings in ways other than in relation to measurement. For example, in a treatment study, we should be concerned that the treatment was delivered in a consistent and repeatable way. If HCPs offered a treatment to different patients in different ways, or to the same patient in different ways at different times, we should have difficulty in claiming that the patient group had really received the treatment we stipulated, and, in consequence, would have less confidence in asserting that any improvements had been the result of the treatment. Note that we are not thinking here of the HCP's natural desire to make treatment individualised to patients. Rather, we are suggesting that if the treatment offered was noticeably and significantly different from one patient to another, difficulties would arise. Indeed, we might argue whether it was, in fact, the same treatment in all cases.

Reliability of measures

Nevertheless, reliability in research is overwhelmingly an issue of measurement, and the reliability of measures is generally examined in terms of whether different raters can use a particular scale and get similar results from it with the same patients. The criteria for judging how similar these results need to be are largely a matter of consensus, and are typically agreed using statistical procedures, but, broadly speaking, we would like raters to agree on their ratings of a patient on somewhere around 80% of occasions. A similar rate of agreement would be expected if the same rater were to rate the same patient on successive occasions (provided, of course, nothing had changed about the patient during that time). These two elements of reliability are known as inter-rater reliability and test-retest reliability, respectively. Internal consistency is a further dimension of reliability and refers to how far different items in a scale are consistent with each other. There is occasionally debate about whether this is actually an issue of reliability (does the scale measure in a consistent way) or validity (does the scale measure what is says it does). Possibly, there are elements of both, because relatedness of items is both a sign of consistency and coherence, and coherence is an important feature of construct validity.

Validity of measures

In measurement, validity refers to whether or not an instrument measures what it claims to. For example, it would be perfectly *reliable* to use heart rate as a measure of anxiety (heart rate is a consistent and repeatable measure), but not necessarily valid (heart rate is raised in many states other than anxiety, like excitement).

Construct validity is one aspect of validity and measures the degree to which a measure relates to some underlying theoretical construct. This is why, as we saw at the end of the previous section, coherence is an important aspect of validity. A measure should be coherent if it is related to a single underlying construct.

Convergent validity refers to the extent to which a measure is related to other measures of a similar construct, whilst divergent validity examines how far it is different from measures which do not examine a similar construct. Predictive validity refers to how accurately a measure can predict behavioural or other outcomes. We might, for example, use an IQ test to predict people's outcomes in a more complex and varied series of tests of intellectual performance (examinations, pieces of assessed work, folios of experience). The ability of the test to predict their performance on these would be an indication of the strength of its predictive values. In a similar way, *concurrent* validity compares a test with some gold standard criterion, but would not include the notion of prediction. These four elements of validity are conceptually very similar.

Content validity is somewhat different in that it refers to the extent to which a measure comprehensively reflects the areas of content it aims to examine. For example, a test of English language ability which tested only punctuation would have poor content validity, because we would all agree there are many other domains of English language ability (spelling, grammar, creative use of imagery and so on).

The weakest form of validity of a measure is face validity, which basically asks whether, on the face of it, the measure appears to measure what it claims to. Face validity can be assessed by, for example, asking a panel of experts (especially patients, carers or other people with whom we expect the eventual measure to be used) whether they feel a scale seems to measure what it purports to. However, this is problematic because experts are fallible, their attention to all elements of the measure may be biased and they may well be unaware of technical elements of a measure which might affect its validity.

Conclusion

The construction of measures which possess good validity and reliability is a difficult, technical and time-consuming process. The same is true, in a more general sense, of the assurance of validity and reliability in quantitative research studies as a whole. For that reason, we can only really scratch the surface in this chapter. With regard to the consideration of reliability and validity in research studies, these issues crop up again in Chapters 15–17, as they are intimately associated with the construction of different quantitative approaches. With regard to the construction of reliable and valid measures, this in particular is a highly technical undertaking, but those of you who are interested will find good starting points in some of the websites below.

Review questions

What different approaches to sampling are mainly used in quantitative research?

Why are these preferred by quantitative researchers?

What are the different types of reliability and validity?

How are reliability and validity related to instruments such as questionnaires?

Exercise

Get hold of a copy of a commonly used questionnaire or other measure. As an example, the Hospital Anxiety and Depression Scale (HADS) is widely used to assess psychological distress in non-psychiatric settings and can be accessed (not for distribution – private study only) at http://www.eardoctor.org/pdf/ Hospital%20Anxiety%20and%20Depression%20Scale.pdf

Ask yourself what the face validity of this questionnaire is. Does it seem to you to adequately investigate what it claims to? If you want, you can then go on to look at studies which have attempted to establish other aspects of the scale's validity and reliability.

Reference

Polgar, S. and Thomas, S.A. (1997) *Introduction to Research in the Health Sciences.* Melbourne: Churchill Livingstone.

Further reading

Burns, N. and Grove, S.K. (2004) *The Practice of Nursing Research*, 5th edn. Philadelphia: Saunders.

Websites

http://chiron.valdosta.edu/whuitt/col/intro/valdgn.html

http://www.socialresearchmethods.net/kb/sampling.php

Cause and Effect, Hypothesis Testing and Estimation

Key points

- Assertions about cause and effect are probabilistic, not definitive.
- We make cause–effect predictions in daily life.
- Cause–effect predictions in healthcare research are the same as those in daily life.
- Quantitative researchers are concerned with independent variables, dependent variables and intervening variables.
- Researchers manipulate independent variables, observe any changes to dependent variables and attempt to account for intervening variables.
- Hypotheses are explicit statements of the predicted relationship between independent and dependent variables.
- Directional hypotheses are made only when there is reason to think a relationship operates only in one direction.
- Adequate statistical power is essential to the safe acceptance of the null hypothesis.
- Hypothesis testing is an all-or-nothing statement of relatedness, but estimation emphasises the extent of a relationship.

Research for Evidence-Based Practice in Healthcare, Second edition, by Robert Newell and Philip Burnard
© 2011 Robert Newell and Philip Burnard

Introduction

The examination of cause and effect is one of the most misunderstood concepts in healthcare research. It has been characterised, variously as mechanistic, unrealistic and over-simple. However, all these assertions about examining cause and effect are themselves based on a version of cause and effect testing and the methods employed to do it (most notably, the randomised controlled trial) which are quite different from those actually practiced by quantitative researchers. Specifically, those who reject methods which seek to establish cause and effect usually do so because they assume that quantitative researchers are claiming the right to a single, definitive answer.

However, this is not so. In fact, quantitative researchers are at pains, in their writing, their research methods and even their statistical procedures (which are all about *probability* not fact) to recognise that their answers to cause and effect questions are always simply the most likely answer *given the current state of our knowledge*. It is explicitly acknowledged that many different factors influence cause and effect relationships, and that not all of them can be controlled or even identified. The best that can be achieved is to be as careful as possible in taking account of as many factors that we *can* control or perceive. As a consequence, it is never claimed that a certain intervention (say, a certain wound care procedure) is *always* the approach of choice for a particular patient problem (a pressure ulcer), only that it is *most likely* to be effective. The habit, amongst many researchers and clinicians, of describing a particular intervention as effective is merely a shorthand for this expression of a likely relationship between a given cause (e.g. treatment) and effect (e.g. patient improvement). This habit has probably given rise to considerable misunderstanding of the nature of scientific 'fact' in quantitative research.

> ### Issues of cause and effect are never definitively answered
>
> Describing a treatment as effective is a shorthand for saying it is *most likely* to be effective, given the current state of our knowledge. It is always acknowledged that there are many influencing factors that cannot be known.

Cause and effect relationships in daily life

Nevertheless, quantitative researchers do say that we live in a cause–effect world. With all the qualifications noted above, it really is contended that, by and large, doing certain things has consequences for patient care and that these can be reliably demonstrated time and time again. However, this is not a stance which is peculiar to quantitative researchers in particular, or even to researchers in general. In Chapter 6, we showed how sampling is a normal everyday activity carried out by all of us. Exactly the same is true for the assessment of cause and effect relationships. Awareness of cause and effect is basic to human life, and, arguably, to the survival of all life. For example, at the level of the other animal species, it is well demonstrated that organisms recognise and avoid aversive stimuli (e.g. pain, loud noises). This is a simple recognition of cause and effect relationships – performing such and such an activity leads to (causes) pain or discomfort and is therefore best avoided.

In our own lives, we make such decisions all the time. Every morning I open my window and look at the sky. If it is cloudy, I predict that it will rain and take an umbrella with me to the station. In doing so, I am making a cause–effect prediction: 'The presence of dark clouds results in rain'. Now, strictly speaking, clouds do not *cause* rain, but I am unaware of the actual processes which do and would, in any case, be unable to measure them without sophisticated equipment. This does not matter, because it is merely an issue of measurement. From my point of view, I have repeatedly tested the assertion that certain kinds of cloudy skies are followed by rain, and this had led to my making the cause–effect link. Nor does it matter if, on a particular occasion, I am proved wrong. What matters is that, most of the time, this cause–effect relationship holds true. Indeed, if it did not, I would soon stop making this prediction and stop carrying my umbrella. I would then be responding to a criterion I had set for myself according to which I would regard my prediction as having been verified or falsified. This brings us again to the notion that cause and effect relationships are almost always *probabilistic*. I also will try to take into account other aspects of the weather (did it rain yesterday, what kind of shape are the clouds, how dark are they, what is the temperature) which, according to my level of knowledge, I will include in my assessment of the likelihood of rain today. This leads us to the assertion that cause and effect predictions are *complex*. This is recognised just as much in research as it is in this everyday example, and we certainly do not expect healthcare research to be less complicated than our everyday decision making.

Cause–effect is part of daily life

In everyday life, we make cause–effect predictions all the time. In doing this, we recognise that we are making probability predictions. Often, we take many complex issues into consideration in making such predictions in important as well as mundane situations. Strangely, we have no problem in doing so – only when this kind of decision is applied to our research or clinical work do people see this as problematic.

Examining cause and effect in healthcare

Therefore, the kinds of cause and effect predictions we make in healthcare can be just as rich, probabilistic and complex as those we make intuitively in everyday life. The methods used to tease out these complexities are often painstaking and complex because, in research, we want to ensure that the processes we have used to arrive at our decisions are transparent to all, in a way which we do not have to do with our own everyday decisions. We want to do this so that others can scrutinise and criticise our work with a clear understanding of what we have done and why we have done it. If necessary, we want to attempt to replicate our work (repeat it using exactly the same methods in a different context). This has given rise to a formal language, which is perhaps unfortunate, but is no different than the verbal shorthand health professionals use to communicate rapidly with each other. The actual processes are little different from the way in which we, as a society, have arrived at our shared knowledge that dark clouds are usually followed by rain.

Variables

In asserting and testing cause–effect relationships, we are basically describing and predicting relationships between *variables*. Variables are any entities in the world which are not fixed, but are subject to change. There are three types of variables to concern us: *independent variables*, *dependent variables* and *intervening variables*. The independent variable is the thing which we, as researchers, vary or *manipulate* in some way. Usually, this is a treatment of some sort. So, if we give one group of patients a relaxation exercise prior to surgery and give another group a premedication sedative, this difference in treatment is the independent variable. It is said to vary over two levels (relaxation and premedication). If we introduce a further group (treatment as normal), the independent variable will then vary over three levels. The use of the word 'level' does not, however, imply that one treatment is more valuable than another, and the term *experimental condition* is sometimes used interchangeably with level. Thus, relaxation, premedication and treatment as normal are three different experimental conditions in the above example.

Levels and conditions – the same, but different

Strictly speaking, levels and conditions are not the same. For example, if we tested two interacting independent variables (exercise regime and intensity of exercise), we could have several levels of each variable: regime (running versus circuit training); intensity (half an hour daily versus an hour every 2 days). So, each variable here consists of two levels. There are four conditions (half an hour daily running, hour bi daily running, half an hour daily circuit, hour bi daily circuit). So, levels refer only to different conditions within a single variable, whilst conditions can be used to describe levels across conditions! Remember, all this is just jargon. It is useful to know the language, so that you can better understand written reports, but it does not materially affect the actual conducting of research.

By contrast with the independent variable, the dependent variable is not manipulated by the researcher. Instead, changes in this variable are regarded as being dependent on the action of the independent variable. In the example above, one possible dependent variable might be patient anxiety, and we would expect the amount of anxiety to differ between the three levels of the independent variable. If this turned out to be the case, we would conclude that these differences were the result of or, *dependent* upon, the actions of the different levels of the independent variable. This is the essence of the investigation of cause–effect relationships in quantitative research.

The relationship between independent and dependent variables

Changes which we measure in the *dependent variable* are regarded as the result of (*dependent on*) our manipulations of the independent variable. In clinical practice, this is like concluding that changes in patient well-being are the result of treatment.

Now, you will readily appreciate that many other things besides the independent variable might affect the patient's anxiety. For example, some patients might have had more experience of surgery than others, might be constitutionally more anxious, or might receive more human attention in one experimental condition than another. These potential sources of bias are discussed in Chapter 13. In examining cause and effect, these sources of bias are called intervening or *confounding* variables. They potentially intervene between the action of the independent variable on the dependent variable and therefore confound our ability to be confident in the existence of a cause and effect relationship. This is exactly the same situation as in the earlier description of my assertion of a cause–effect relationship between dark clouds and rain. There are many other factors which might account for the result, other than the assumed cause. As we shall see in Chapters 15, 16 and 17, much quantitative research which investigates cause–effect relationships is concerned with trying to eliminate or control for the effect of these intervening variables. This is because intervening variables undermine our confidence that a cause–effect relationship has been demonstrated by weakening internal validity (see Chapter 13).

In summary, researchers interested in cause–effect relationships seek to establish these by examining the relationship between the independent variable and the dependent variable, whilst minimising the influence of any intervening variables.

Hypotheses

These relationships are usually expressed as explicit statements of the predicted influence of the independent variable on the dependent variable, and these explicit statements are called hypotheses. Hypotheses are always very specific, but are usually based on general ideas of supposed relationships between entities in the world. Hypotheses may be derived from broad theories about how the world is supposed to work, from previous studies or speculations, and often from descriptive studies or qualitative approaches which have not sought to establish cause–effect relationships. Hypotheses are always framed as predictive statements about what is expected to happen, rather than as questions. Research questions are generally broader in compass than are hypotheses. So, a typical hypothesis with regard to our preoperative anxiety study would be: 'Patients will experience greater preoperative anxiety after receiving a premedication injection than after receiving instruction in relaxation techniques' NOT 'Do patients experience greater anxiety after receiving a premedication injection than after receiving instruction in relaxation techniques?'

Whilst this is a minor stylistic point, the issue of precise specification is more important because precision helps the researcher to *operationalise* the research question in a way which is measurable and not open to debate or imprecision. The conditions which need to be fulfilled for the hypothesis to be supported are clearly stated. The essential elements in a hypothesis should be the independent variable and its experimental conditions, the dependent variable, and the conditions under which the relationship between the variables is asserted to exist. So, in the above example, the independent variable and its experimental conditions are relaxation/premedication, the independent variable is anxiety and the conditions are 'preoperative'. Notice that we have not stated how great the difference is required to be or how it should be measured. Indeed, Burns and Grove (2004) argue that precise statement of measurement conditions is *not* required, because this is an issue related to samples, whilst hypotheses are designed to assert proposed relationships between populations (see Chapter 6). A counter argument is that adequacy of a hypothesis rests in large part upon its ability to state the necessary and sufficient conditions required for testing of a cause–effect relationship. Accordingly, if a statement of measurement helps with this, it should be included, but if it does not, it may be omitted.

Experimental and null hypotheses

Typically, an *experimental hypothesis* is a statement of what might be expected to occur if the experimental condition in an experiment differed from the control condition, or, in situations where two different treatments are compared, if a difference existed between those two treatments. Our hypothesis in the preoperative anxiety example is an experimental hypothesis. A statement of an expectation of *no* difference is called a *null hypothesis* and, in the same example would be stated as follows: 'That there will be no difference in preoperative anxiety between patients receiving premedication and those receiving instruction in relaxation training'.

Researchers typically speak of rejecting the null hypothesis and accepting the experimental hypothesis when there is a difference between the experimental groups (in this case, relaxation and premedication), and accepting the null hypothesis and rejecting the experimental hypothesis when there is not. In the physical sciences, it is more usual to speak chiefly of accepting or rejecting the null hypothesis, whilst in the social sciences it has become more normal to speak of rejecting or accepting the experimental hypothesis. However, this is largely a verbal distinction rather than an actual procedural difference. The important issue is that, in each case, both experimental hypothesis and null hypothesis are clearly defined and mutually exclusive. In an experiment, there can never be a situation where both the experimental hypothesis and its corresponding null hypothesis can be accepted.

Whilst the verbal distinction we have just described is largely a matter of academic debate rather than practical importance, a somewhat similar distinction *is* important. This is the difference between *predicting* the experimental hypothesis and predicting the null hypothesis. By and large, it is poor research practice to make a prediction of no difference between two groups. Even if we believed that the two treatments (relaxation and premedication) were likely to have a similar effect on patients' anxiety, a prediction of the null hypothesis does not, in hypothesis testing, allow us to assess adequately the similarity or difference between two treatments. This is because there could be many causes of our failing to find differences between the treatments other than their similarity. For example, there might be differences between the patients in each treatment group, or there might be insufficient patients to show a statistical difference. In other words, failing to find a difference between two things is not the same as finding they are alike, and the null hypothesis is merely a statement of finding no difference. Where we actually want to demonstrate that two treatments are similar, or *equivalent*, we have to construct an *experimental hypothesis* which adequately captures what we mean by similarity, rather than simply predicting the null hypothesis.

Directional and non-directional hypotheses

The patient anxiety study we constructed a hypothesis for above gives an example of what is called a *directional hypothesis*. We predict not only that the two treatments will have different effects, but that one will yield better results (lower anxiety) than the other. In other words, we state the direction in which we believe the results will go – patients receiving relaxation will experience *less* anxiety than those receiving premedication. However, we should only construct directional hypotheses where we have good reason to suppose the results are likely to go in a particular direction. In this example, it may be that a directional hypothesis is not appropriate. Can we really be confident that relaxation will be better than premedication, rather than worse, and if so why? Unless we can bring evidence to bear to justify constructing a directional hypothesis (whether from theory, clinical experience or earlier pilot studies), a *non-directional hypothesis* may well be more appropriate. Such hypotheses merely predict that the experimental groups will be different, not the direction of that difference. For our preoperative patients, a non-directional hypothesis would be: 'Preoperative anxiety will be different in patients receiving relaxation instruction and those receiving premedication'.

There are, however, two very good reasons for constructing directional hypotheses when it is possible to do so. First, hypotheses are often based on previous knowledge or theory, and we should aim for as stringent a test of such theory or knowledge as possible. This will often lead to directional predictions, which are precisely linked to the theory they attempt to test. Second, directional hypotheses are much more sensitive, for statistical reasons, and so are more likely to detect differences between the experimental groups when these are present.

Grounds for rejecting and accepting hypotheses

Hypotheses are accepted or rejected purely on statistical grounds (see Chapter 20) and these grounds are probabilistic, both mathematically and in the everyday way we described earlier in this chapter. As a result, there will be times when we mistakenly reject the null hypothesis when it is true and accept it when it is false. These errors are called *type I errors* and *type II errors*, respectively, and may result from statistical and methodological difficulties. The statistical issues are discussed in Chapter 20, and some commentators describe type I and type II error (particularly type I) almost entirely in statistical terms. In one sense, this is correct, because the decision to accept or reject a hypothesis is indeed made on statistical grounds. However, many methodological issues (e.g. poor measurement, poor allocation of patients to one or other experimental condition, insufficient participants) contribute to the data on which statistical tests are performed.

Power to reject the experimental hypothesis

Lack of sufficient participants to show a difference between the experimental conditions is a particularly pressing issue in healthcare research, where numbers of participants are often very small indeed. In such cases, the grounds for rejecting the experimental hypothesis are often very slim. This is because such small group studies, which are said to be *underpowered*, are susceptible to subject variability (the natural tendency for individual participants to vary in their personal attributes and the tendency for those attributes to contribute to their response to manipulation of the independent variable).

Whilst random allocation can, to a certain degree, iron out any systematic variation on participant characteristics, it cannot account for unsystematic variation in these characteristics. This is important because the apparent response of a person to a treatment is essentially a combination of their own individual characteristics and their actual response to the treatment. In our preoperative anxiety example, randomisation can, to a large extent, get over the problem of having lots of naturally anxious people in one treatment condition and not the other. However, randomisation cannot help in situations where participants in each group vary greatly on the measure of treatment effectiveness (in this case, reduced anxiety). High levels of this *intra-subject variability* can obscure effects of the independent variable because the contribution made by individual variation to the variations in scores between the groups is large in comparison to the variation accounted for by the different treatments. As a simple example, suppose that, in our group of preoperative patients, their anxiety varied on average by about two points on a 1–10 scale. At the same time, we know that a two-point decrease in anxiety is likely to be clinically important. The problem for us is to tease out whether observing such a decrease is the result of natural fluctuations in patient scores or the action of the different treatments.

There are several solutions for this problem, all of which are said to increase the power of a study to detect treatment differences where these are present. First, we may select a more homogeneous patient group, so that their individual fluctuation interferes less with the treatment effect. Second, we may choose a measure which is more sensitive to treatment effects. Third, we may set a higher treatment *effect size* (the size of difference between the groups we regard as clinically important), although we would need a good clinical reason to do so, not simply a desire to increase the power of the study. Finally, and most commonly, we can increase the number of participants in the study. This works because larger groups typically have less intra-subject variability, and so the effect of the independent variable is more easily seen, as there is less interference from subject variability.

The power of a study is now almost always decided at the planning phase, by performing a *power calculation* based on what we know from other studies of the likely effect size of the treatment and the degree of variability amongst participants. Knowing or being able to estimate these two things enables us to calculate the number of participants needed to stand a reasonable chance (usually a 9 out of 10 or 90% chance) of detecting treatment differences where these are present. Generally speaking, it is inappropriate to take much notice of underpowered studies which result in a rejection of the experimental hypothesis. For a full discussion of power, see Kraemer and Thiemann (1987).

Underpowered studies rarely produce valid rejection of the experimental hypothesis

Underpowered studies which result in a rejection of the experimental hypothesis are likely to be misleading. This is because, in such studies, the individual differences between participants account for so much of the variation in the group as a whole (both groups) that an intervention would need to be extremely effective in order to override this and show a difference between the groups. This would be fine if only *extremely effective* interventions were useful. However, even an intervention which makes a small difference is often important. Underpowered studies miss this difference because of the impact of individual variability on the overall amount of variability observed.

Estimation

In testing hypotheses, we are concerned with making a single, categorical decision – to either accept or reject the null hypothesis. However, it has been argued that many outcomes in healthcare (as well as in related fields such as psychology and sociology) are not well expressed in terms of such an all-or-nothing cut-off. We use a statistical significance level of <5% (1 time in 20) as appropriate grounds for rejecting the null hypothesis. If the level is *actually* 5%, this is not generally taken as grounds on which to reject the null hypothesis – if it hits the post, it is not a goal. Many researchers regard this position as intuitively wrong. There are, after all, many things one wants to know about a football match other than the number of goals scored. Similarly, in health research, there may well be many measures, or *estimates*, of important variations in results, other than the simple recording of a probability score (p value). The estimation of parameters approach reflects these concerns.

For example, rather than testing the hypothesis that people will sleep better on average with relaxation exercises than sleeping tablets, estimation allows us to specify how much improvement we think will be important and test how likely it is that such a level of improvement, if found in our sample group, is an adequate reflection of likely changes in the theoretical population from which that sample has been drawn. So, in our study of sleep, estimation tells us the likely parameters for the population score. If our sample score (usually, the mean) lies between these two parameters, we can be confident that this score is an adequate refection of the population score, or, to be more precise, of *a* population score somewhere between those two parameters. The narrower the distance between those parameters, the more accurate a reflection the sample score is of the population. By and large, the larger our sample, the smaller the space between the population parameters will be.

In treatment comparison studies, we often apply estimation to the *difference* scores between two groups, and the additional information the estimation approach gives us is that it tells us how far the sample difference score reflects the difference between the two theoretical populations (in our example, *all* people with sleep problems who might receive either relaxation or sleeping pills). To return to our football image, hypothesis testing tells us whether a shot has hit the goal, whilst estimation also tells us how far apart the goalposts were. Clearly, a shot has to be much more accurate to hit a smaller goal.

Review questions

Why aren't cause–effect relationships definitive?

What is the difference between the null hypothesis and the experimental hypothesis?

What is meant by the terms independent variable, dependent variable and intervening variable?

What is the main problem with underpowered studies?

What is the difference between hypothesis testing and estimation?

Exercises

(1) Using the preoperative anxiety example as a model, construct a hypothesis to investigate an area of your own clinical practice. Remember to specify the independent and dependent variables precisely.

(2) Consider the comparative merits of hypothesis testing and estimation in answering clinical research questions. Consult Altman *et al.* (2001), second edition of the classic text on this matter.

(3) Access the following site: http://www.dssresearch.com/ toolkit/spcalc/power_a2.asp

Put in some imaginary values for mean, standard deviation and sample size for each of the two samples (you can think of the two samples as being people having two different treatments of your choice [or treatment and no treatment], and think of mean and standard deviation as giving measures of the amount of individual variability in each of the groups). Once you have entered these values, hit the *Calculate sample size* button to get the power. Now, try changing the values. You should see that, as the standard deviations (representing individual variability) get bigger, you need more people in the study to get the same level of power. Also, for any given values of the mean and standard deviation, altering the sample size alters the power (the smaller the sample, the lower the power).

References

Altman, D.G., Machin, D., Bryant, T.N. and Gardner, M.J. (2001) *Statistics with Confidence*. London: BMJ Books.

Burns, N. and Grove, S.K. (2004) *The Practice of Nursing Research*, 5th edn. Philadelphia: Saunders.

Thompson, D. and Martin, C. (2001) *Design and Analysis of Clinical Nursing Research Studies*. London: Routledge.

Further reading

Kraemer, H.C. and Thiemann, S. (1987) *How Many Subjects? Statistical Power Analysis in Research*. London: Sage.

Newell, R. (1994) Variables and hypotheses. *Nurse Researcher*, 1(4), 37–47.

Websites

http://www.dssresearch.com/toolkit/spcalc/power_a2.asp

http://www.shef.ac.uk/content/1/c6/06/59/35/Scope%20tutorial%204.pdf

15

Experimental and Quasi-Experimental Approaches

Key points

- Experiments consist of three elements: manipulation of the independent variable, use of a control group and random allocation to experimental conditions.
- These three elements allow experiments to claim a high degree of internal validity.
- Quasi-experimental designs use a similar *general* approach to true experiments but control and/or random assignment may be missing.
- Repeated measures approaches use the same participants for all experimental conditions.
- Repeated measures approaches are vulnerable to order effects.
- Order effects may be reduced by counterbalancing.
- Independent groups designs use different participants for different experimental conditions.
- Independent groups designs without randomisation are vulnerable to differences in participant characteristics (subject variability).
- Matched pairs designs match participants on important variables to combat subject variability.
- Factorial designs study interactions between several different independent variables.

Research for Evidence-Based Practice in Healthcare, Second edition, by Robert Newell and Philip Burnard
© 2011 Robert Newell and Philip Burnard

Introduction

Experimental research is a broad expression which covers so-called 'true experiments' plus a range of approaches which are not, strictly speaking, true experiments, but similar approaches which lack certain aspects of the true experiment. What all these approaches, including true experiments, share is the deliberate manipulation of the independent variable and the systematic observation of changes in the dependent variable (see Chapter 14). The aim of all forms of experimental research is to reduce the effects of bias on the observation of this relationship between the independent and dependent variables. The greater the level of control of this possible bias, the greater the confidence we can have in asserting a cause and effect relationships.

True experiments

In true experiments, the level of control over bias is higher than in any other type of research, and, therefore, our confidence in asserting cause–effect relationships can be equally high. As we noted in the previous chapter, such assertions are always probabilistic, but, within this constraint, true experiments allow us the greatest certainty that changes in the dependent variable are consequences of differences between levels of the independent variable, rather than of uncontrolled variations such as participant or environmental variation. Experiments achieve this through a combination of three aspects of experimental design: manipulation of the independent variable; use of a control group; random allocation to different experimental conditions (levels of the independent variable).

Manipulation is the most basic feature of experimental research, including true experiments. We saw in the previous chapter that it is a conscious decision of the researcher, in experimental research, to vary the levels of the independent variable. This immediately gives the researcher great control. It is quite possible for us to select different *naturally occurring* levels of an independent variable, but this is not an experiment or quasi-experiment. To return for a moment to the example of preoperative anxiety used in Chapter 14, you will recall we gave patients either premedication of relaxation exercises. It would have been equally possible, for example, to take patients from different clinical settings, some of which offered premedication whilst others offered relaxation. However, as you will appreciate, the level of control over levels of the independent variable would immediately be decreased.

In this kind of situation (sometimes referred to, confusingly, as a *natural experiment*) we know nothing about, for example, what different sorts of premedication might be in use, what different types of relaxation might be used, how patients might be selected, what other factors might be operating in the clinical settings, and so on. Thus, in the absence of manipulation of the independent variable, the opportunity for bias is immediate and considerable and, as a result, the confidence with which we can assert cause–effect relationships is greatly decreased. Some writers (e.g. Roe and Webb, 1998) suggest that selection of different groups of people on the basis of different characteristics they already possess (e.g. men and women) and then comparing their responses is a form of manipulation. Whilst this kind of procedure is entirely appropriate (and we will discuss it in our examination of non-experimental research in Chapter 18), it is not, strictly speaking, a manipulation of the independent variable. It is simply another example of a group observational comparison of naturally occurring variation in the independent variable. After all, we cannot decide who is male and who is female. This point is of more than just academic importance because of the reduction in purity of the cause–effect relationship, because our male and female participants may be different in many ways other than their gender. Only where some clearly identifiable aspect of gender could be isolated would this approach approximate to a true experiment in terms of its ability to demonstrate cause–effect relationships. Certainly, no study which contained such an approach could be described as an experiment, because it would, in any case lack the random assignment characteristic of experiments. We cannot randomly assign people to gender (or to any other personal characteristic).

The second aspect of the experiment is the control of unwanted sources of variability, the *intervening* or *confounding variables* we discussed in the previous chapter. This often involves the use of a control group, and this is an extension of the notion of manipulation of the independent variable. Essentially, the researcher tries to control the environment in such a way that the only thing which differs between the groups involved in the study is the independent variable. In so doing, the researcher must account for both the subject and environmental variability we discussed in Chapter 14. Using a control group is an important contribution to this because it is a very good way of controlling for subject variability (see the discussion of how different designs do this later in this chapter) and of creating a controlled environment in which the independent variable can be tightly specified. In our preoperative anxiety example, the researcher can potentially allocate similar patients to each experimental condition and so design the environment that there is little difference between the two conditions other than the offering of either premedication or relaxation. For example, some circumstances which might affect the response to the two interventions include nature of the operation being performed, experience of the ward, theatre and recovery staff, type of premedication offered, prior patient experience of hospitals and operations. Although it is difficult in practice to control for these different circumstances, this is the ideal to which control in experiments aspires. The greater the extent to which a researcher is able to exert such experimental control, the greater the *internal validity* of the experiment.

Randomisation is, in many ways, a particular aspect of control: the control of subject variability. In non-randomised studies, there is always the possibility that systematic bias in subject selection may creep into the process of allocation to one or other experimental condition. Participants selected in other ways (e.g. age, educational background, gender, postcode, convenience) may differ greatly from each other in ways we are unaware of but which may affect their performance. Although not perfect, randomisation to one or other experimental condition minimises the likelihood of these unwanted sources of subject variability interfering with the effect of the independent variable. The concept of randomisation is discussed in more detail in Chapter 17, which considers the randomised controlled trial (the application of the experiment to clinical studies), which has emerged as the key procedure for decreasing the effects of subject variability in healthcare research studies.

One aspect of subject variability which randomisation cannot control so well is unsystematic variability where the level of variability between subjects in terms of their response to the action of the independent variability is very wide. For control of this, increasing subject numbers is the most usual way, as described in our discussion of power in Chapter 14.

Quasi-experimental designs

Quasi-experimental designs, as the name suggests, use a similar *general* approach to true experiments, in that manipulation, control and random assignment are all of importance. However, whilst manipulation is always present in quasi-experimental approaches, control, randomisation or both may be missing. You will occasionally see definitions of quasi-experimental design which suggest that both manipulation and control must be present but most researchers agree that only the presence of manipulation is required for a study to count as quasi-experimental. Now, it may seem, at first, glance, that if a study is non-randomised then control is, by definition, lacking. This is not so, however, because we can systematically allocate to different levels of the independent variable in non-random ways (e.g. by gender, by health status and so on). Conversely, a study can be randomised but still lack control. Even in the presence of a control group, it may be impossible to adequately isolate key components of the environment in a way which results in the independent variable being the only thing to vary between the groups.

These missing elements give rise to the lower strength of relationship between the independent and dependent variables in quasi-experimental approaches. However, quasi-experimental approaches have distinct advantages, particularly in healthcare, where random allocation may be difficult to organise or considered unethical, and where the complex, changing nature of the environment of care may make the elimination of confounding variables impossible. The reduction in internal validity may be more than offset by the practical advantages of quasi-experimental approaches. Moreover, there is a potential increase in external validity in studies which contain some element of confounding, because such complex environments are closer to the real world. Indeed, randomised controlled trials are regularly criticised precisely because of this lack of conformity to the messy real world of healthcare (see Chapter 17).

For the remainder of this chapter, we will consider several key approaches to quasi-experimental research as they relate to healthcare, and explore their strengths and weaknesses with regard to the way they deal with threats to internal validity.

Repeated measures approaches

This comparatively simple approach will be intuitively familiar to many HCPs because it is in many ways similar to what we do when we observe the health status of patients in clinical practice[1]. In repeated measures studies, sometimes called *before–after* studies, randomisation and a separate control group are both usually lacking, although other aspects of environmental and subject variability can be controlled. The defining feature of the repeated measures study is that each participant receives each level of the independent variable. The researcher may, however, decide on such issues as the order in which participants receive each level. Thus, there is some element of manipulation. As an example, in a group of people with constipation, a dietician might measure frequency of bowel motions, then offer the entire group of participants an intervention for constipation (say, bran or other bulking agents), then measure frequency of bowel motions again. The two repeated measures represent two different levels of the independent variable – no treatment (baseline) and treatment (bran). Naturally, in this simplest form of repeated measures study, no randomisation is possible, because the baseline phase could not easily come after the treatment phase. In the absence of a period of baseline measurement, it is doubtful that we have any meaningful manipulation of the independent variable. In our example, this is obvious, because we need a baseline phase from a practical point of view to get a measure of frequency of bowel motions. Supposing, however, we gave our participants a self-report measure which asked them to rate their bowel movement

Baseline – measure – bran – measure – bowel retraining – measure – bran +
bowel retraining – measure

Figure 15.1 Repeated measures design.

frequency retrospectively, then gave them a similar measure at the end
of the treatment phase. This looks at first like a repeated measures design quasi-experiment, but it is not. This is because it is quite false to say
that the pre-measure represents a no-treatment level of the independent
variable. After all, what we have is a retrospective account of a period
of time when we have no idea what the patients were doing with regard to their bowel habit. They may, for example, have taken aperients,
or even bran itself. They may also have had physical illnesses which affected their bowel function. Now, whilst this kind of variability affects
all research, including quasi-experiments and experiments, this is not
the point at issue here. Rather, without baseline, we are not manipulating the independent variable, simply observing (somewhat unsystem-
atically) naturally occurring variability during the pre-treatment phase.

We could add to this simplest form of repeated measures design almost infinitely by substituting further treatments consecutively. For example, we could substitute bowel retraining for bran. We could also
add treatments, offering bran and bowel retraining together, once again
to the same group of participants (see Figure 15.1). We could also introduce further periods of no treatment (control phases) between each
active intervention.

Interrupted time series analysis

When we add several data collection points between different levels of
the independent variable (treatment or control), we are using an *interrupted time-series design* in which statistical comparisons are made between different time points in a treatment-control sequence. Between
the introduction of each new intervention, there are several time points
at which measurements are taken.

Simplest form of interrupted time series analysis

C1, C2, C3, C4, C5, C6 – T1, T2, T3, T4, T5, T6 – C7, C8, C9, C10, C11,
C12
C = Control
T = Treatment

Each new phase represents a further level of the independent variable, and a degree of randomisation can be included, in terms of the order in which each level is offered, greatly strengthening the design. Statistical comparisons are made between each consecutive set of measures, in much the same way as we might monitor patients' responses to a series of different interventions in a clinical context.

There are numerous advantages to the repeated measures design. Notice that, in the above example, we do not need to add extra participants to add extra experimental conditions. This can be particularly advantageous where participants are hard to find, as in a complaint which is comparatively rare. Also, there is typically no subject variability in repeated measures designs, because the same participants take part in each experimental condition. Thus, systematic subject bias between the groups is entirely avoided. Even where subject variability is large, repeated measures designs are still helpful, because the overall number of subjects required to reduce this to an acceptable level will always be considerably less than in designs where different subjects receive different levels of the independent variable. Finally, where further measurement points are added (as in time series analysis) there may be increased control of maturation effects (uncontrolled variation over time) because of the ability to examine trends in the data and use statistical procedures to account for these. In summary, repeated measures designs are very good at accounting for subject variability because participants effectively act as their own controls.

However, control of environmental sources of bias is less good. Even though subjects receive all levels of the independent variable, they are still open to the effects of confounding differences between the different levels, and similar attempts at control must be made as in true experiments. One particular problem with repeated measures designs is the presence of practice effects and other carry-over effects between the conditions. In our constipation example, we might easily find that offering bran exerted such a powerful influence that subsequent offering of bowel retraining contributed little to the group's bowel motion frequency. In such a case, a return to baseline might offer a 'wash-out' period during which the effects of the first intervention would have a chance to wear off before the next intervention was offered. However, had we offered bowel retraining first, it might prove very difficult to offer such a washout period, because it is extremely difficult to 'unlearn' things one has been taught. These sorts of *order effect* can be compelling drawbacks to repeated measures designs in other contexts, too, such as studies of perception or attitude, in which offering one experimental condition primes to participant by facilitating their performance during subsequent conditions or alerting them to the objectives of the research in ways which interfere with its purpose.

Typically, some sort of *counter-balancing* across the conditions is an adequate solution to many order effects, and in health research such

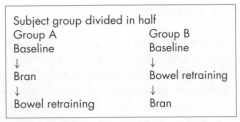

Figure 15.2 Counterbalancing in repeated measures designs.

counterbalancing is usually referred to as a *crossover study*. In this approach, subjects receive all levels of the independent variable, but in different orders (see Figure 15.2). Thus, any bias introduced by order is eliminated. We might further refine this by allocating subjects randomly to one or other of the counterbalanced conditions. Statistical comparisons are made between the pooled results of participants according to condition, but regardless of order. In some designs, a specific statistical adjustment may be made to investigate the impact of order effects on the pooled results. As they lack subject variability across conditions, repeated measures designs typically are more sensitive to effects of the independent variable than is the other major contender in quasi-experimental research, the *independent groups* (or divided groups) design.

Independent groups designs

The true experiment is actually an independent groups design experiment. The only difference between the true experiment and other independent groups designs is that randomisation and/or control are missing. The advantage of the independent groups design over repeated measure designs is that order effects are not an issue, because each participant receives only one level of the independent variable. On the debit side, all the difficulties of subject variability in the true experiment are also present, but accentuated because of the lack of randomisation or other control. However, as we noted earlier, randomisation may be difficult to achieve in many settings. In these settings, where repeated measures studies are impractical (e.g. because issues of order effects cannot be overcome), non-randomised independent groups studies are usually the only practical alternative. Effectively, these are non-randomised control group studies, where we cannot be certain that the experimental and control groups are similar in nature.

Control group time series designs

As we saw in the description of repeated measures designs, sometimes multiple data collection points are possible between the introduction of different levels of the independent variable. Once again, the gain for researchers is the diminution of the risk of chance findings (because there are more data points, which tend to reduce variability in the data), and the ability examine and account for uncontrolled variability.

> **Simple control group time series design**
>
> A1, A2, A3, A4 – T – A5, A6, A7, A8
> B1, B2, B3, B4 – C – B5 B6, B7, B8
> A = Treatment group (bran)
> B = Control group (no bran)

Interrupted time series designs are a potentially powerful investigative approach. We recommend the work of Gene Glass in this area, and an excellent chapter by him on the Arizona State University website stands the test of time and gives a good discussion of issues in time series design from a broad range of health and social care and policy perspectives (http://glass.ed.asu.edu/gene/papers/tsx.pdf).

Matched pairs designs

One way of overcoming subject variability when repeated measures designs or randomisation are not feasible is the use of a *matched pairs* approach, in which pairs of subjects are matched and then allocated to one or other level of the independent variable. The classic example of this is the use of twin studies, but we can match subjects in many ways. Good matching depends on selecting criteria according to which to match them that comprehensively account for elements of subject variability likely to be important in the study in question. In the constipation example, we might well match subjects for age and gender, but this would be very general matching indeed, and would be greatly strengthened if we extended the matching process to take into account, for example, current diet, medical history (particularly of bowel disease), medication, exercise levels. Finally, there is no reason why a matched pairs approach should not be used in a true experiment, with individuals being randomly allocated to one or other experimental condition on a pair-by-pair basis. See Weiss and Klein (2005) for an example of a widely cited recent matched pairs design study in child physiotherapy.

Factorial studies

So far, we have only looked at the investigation of a single independent variable at a time, even though this variable might vary over several levels. Sometimes, however, we want to look at the effects of several independent variables together, to see if and how they interact. To return to the constipation example, we had three levels of a single independent variable (the intervention – no treatment [baseline], bran, bowel retraining). We also noted that we could use additive treatments (bran and bowel retraining together). With this kind of interaction (between bran and bowel retraining) we can continue to use either a repeated measures of independent groups approach, because we are actually just adding a further level to the single independent variable (intervention – now consisting of no treatment [baseline], bran, bowel retraining, bran and bowel retraining together).

However, this is not always possible. Say, we wanted to assess the effects of two different approaches to learning in student radiographers (self-directed study and classroom tuition) on their performance, the effect of time of day during which the approach was delivered, *and* the interaction between these two things. Now, in the first example, we just have one question (which intervention is better?) and one independent variable (intervention), even though one of these interventions consists of two additive treatments. In the second, we are asking three questions (which learning approach gives better performance (regardless of time of day)? Which time of day gives better performance (regardless of learning approach?) Do the different approaches yield different levels of performance if given at different times of day (Is there an interaction between approach and time of delivery?)? Such designs are very powerful because they allow the examination of complex interventions but retain experimental control. The other main contender for examining such complex interventions (which often occur in healthcare) is through correlation (see Chapter 18) which lacks such robustness because it is essentially observational and therefore open to many potential sources of bias.

As you can perhaps see from the previous paragraph, factorial designs are, however, often difficult to conceptualise and organise, but repay the effort because of their ability to examine complex interactions. Figure 15.3 shows a simple graphical way of conceptualising factorial designs. For simplicity, the figure shows a 2 × 2 factorial design. That is, it possesses two independent variables, each varying over two levels. This design allows the examination of one interaction. However, complex factorial designs may contain several independent variables, each varying over several levels, and thus allowing many interactions to be examined.

	Independent variable (IV) 1: learning approach	
Independent variable (IV) 2: time of delivery	Experimental condition 1: IV1 level 1 – Self-directed learning: IV2 level 1 – morning	Experimental condition 2: IV1 level 2 – classroom teaching: IV2 level 2 – morning
	Experimental condition 3: IV1 level 1 – Self-directed learning: IV2 level 2 – evening	Experimental condition 4: IV1 level 2 – classroom teaching: IV2 level 2 – evening

Figure 15.3   Investigation of learning approach and time of delivery.

The example given here consists entirely of independent groups variables. However, it is possible to have some independent variables organised for independent groups and others for repeated measures. For example, in this example, time of day and method of learning could both have been organised as repeated measures variables, perhaps for different teaching topics.

Likewise, teaching topic could have been specified as a further independent variable, creating a 3 × 2 factorial design (three independent variables each varying over two levels) and allowing us to look at three separate effects on performance – Which learning approach gives better performance (regardless of time of day or teaching topic)? Which time of day gives better performance (regardless of learning approach or teaching topic)? Which teaching topic gives better performance (regardless of learning approach or time of day)? We can also look at four different interactions: do the different approaches yield different levels of performance if given at different times of day (Is there an interaction between approach and time of delivery?)? Do the different approaches yield different levels of performance with different teaching topics (Is there an interaction between approach and topic?)? Do the different topics yield different levels of performance if delivered at different times (Is there an interaction between topic and time of delivery?)? Do the different topics yield different levels of performance when delivered with different learning approaches at according to different times of the day (Is there an additive interaction between topic, approach and time of delivery?)?

Conclusion

These approaches to quasi-experimental research designs represent different attempts to solve different threats to the internal validity of a study, whether these arise from bias as a result of subject variability or confounding variables in the environment. In essence, repeated measures designs are particularly strong at eliminating subject variability, whilst independent groups designs are less sensitive to unwanted order effects and can offer a greater level of control. There are numerous variants, particularly to independent groups quasi-experimental designs. Many of these are designed to overcome particular practical constraints, rather than to increase the validity of the design. Interested readers can find details of variants on repeated measures quasi-experimental designs at http://www.socialresearchmethods.net/kb/quasiexp.php.

Matched pairs designs combine many of the strengths of independent groups and repeated measures designs, provided the matching strategy is appropriate to the issue being investigated. Factorial designs may be independent groups, repeated measures or a mix of both, and so are subject to the strengths and weaknesses of these designs. They are the only experimental research approach to investigating complex interactions between different independent variables.

Finally, we noted that true experiments were one form of independent groups design. It should also be noted that greater or less degrees of randomisation can also be introduced into repeated measures designs, matched pairs designs and factorial designs, as can greater levels of control. For example, a factorial design with subjects randomly assigned to each condition of each independent variable and which possesses good use of controls is essentially a form of true experiment, whilst a non-randomised factorial design clearly is not. Similarly, a repeated measures design which randomly assigns the order in which subjects receive different levels of the independent variable *may* be experimental provided control of confounding (e.g., by order effects) is adequate. The more these elements are incorporated into such designs, the more we are justified in saying they appear like true experiments, and, in consequence, the more the cause–effect inferences we draw from them can approach those we might draw from true experiments. Indeed, the general rule is that the greater control of threats to internal validity in a study, the greater confidence we can have in attributing a causal role to the independent variable

Review questions

What are the three necessary components of true experiments?
What differentiates between experimental and quasi-experimental approaches?
What are the strengths and weaknesses of repeated measures and independent groups approaches?

> **Exercise**
>
> Consider the problem of sleep in hospital. Would an experimental approach be able to investigate solutions to this problem? What alternative designs might work?

Endnote

1. See Law *et al.* (2005) for a fairly large scale before–after study in a community setting.

References

Law, M., Majnemer, A., McColl, M.A., Bosch, J., Hanna, S., Wilkins, S., Birch, S., Telford, J. and Stewart, D. (2005) Home and community occupational therapy for children and youth: a before and after study. *Canadian Journal of Occupational Therapy*, 72(5), 289–297.

Roe, B. and Webb, C. (1998) *Research and Development in Clinical Nursing Practice*. London: Taylor & Francis.

Weiss, H.R. and Klein, R. (2005) Improving excellence in scoliosis rehabilitation: a controlled study of matched pairs. *Pediatric Rehabilitation*, 9(3), 190–200.

Further reading

Beck, S.L. (1989) The crossover design in nursing research. *Nursing Research*, 38(5), 291–293

Cook, T. and Campbell, D. (1979) *Quasi-Experimentation: Design and Analysis for Field Settings*. Chicago: Rand McNally.

Field, A. and Hole, G.J. (2002) *How to Design and Report Experiments*. London: Sage.

Shadish, W.R., Cook, T. and Campbell, D.T. (2001) *Experimental and Quasi-Experimental Designs for Generalised Causal Inference*. Boston: Hoghton Mifflin.

Website

http://www.*csulb*.edu/~msaintg/ppa696/696quasi.htm

16

The Single Case Experiment

Key points

- Single case experiments apply experimental methods to treatment of single individuals.
- Single case experiments allow you to do research in the course of clinical practice.
- In AB designs and variants, different interventions are introduced and withdrawn sequentially.
- In multiple baseline designs, responses to different interventions are compared cross-sectionally.
- Systematized measurement is essential to single case experiments.
- Data analysis is often confined to visual inspection of changes in scores.
- Visual inspection can involve examining raw scores, means, levels, trends and latencies.
- Statistical approaches have been developed because interpretation of visual data can be subject to bias.
- Single case experiments have good internal validity but poor external validity.

Research for Evidence-Based Practice in Healthcare, Second edition, by Robert Newell and Philip Burnard
© 2011 Robert Newell and Philip Burnard

What is a single case experimental design?

Single case experiments have rarely been used in healthcare research, apart from occasionally by nurses, psychologists and other professions working in the field of cognitive-behaviour therapy (CBT) (in which discipline the approach has its clinical roots) and in some specialist branches of physiotherapy, occupational therapy and clinical psychology, and so are unlikely to be familiar to you. Moreover, medicine has likewise largely ignored this type of research. This is perhaps surprising, given that both healthcare and medicine have relied heavily in the past on the single case *report* when describing unusual illnesses or patient problems, or when reporting novel attempts at treating such problems. However, the single case experiment is very different from the case report, and is, in many respects, closer to the randomised controlled trial and quasi-experimental methods than to the kind of qualitative, descriptive approach typical in case reports.

The chief distinction between case reports and single case experiments (or single case experimental designs [SCEDs]) is that case reports have no ability to tease out cause and effect relationships. Therefore, any assertions made on the basis of case reports are essentially just that – assertions of possible cause and effect made on the basis of often unsystematic observations of problems and their treatment. Popular and professional healthcare journals contain considerable numbers of such reports, and so they are a familiar way of communicating novel treatment approaches to HCPs.

Unfortunately, HCPs would be unwise to implement the treatments outlined in such case study material without further corroborating evidence of its effectiveness, because of the inherent weakness in case reports of failing to identify the independent, dependent and intervening variables (see Chapter 14). By contrast, SCEDS attempt to specify, identify and control these three key aspects of the examination of cause and effect relationships. In essence, as the name suggests, an SCED is a type of experiment applied to an individual, and seeks to discover whether an intervention or series of interventions are to bring about change in that individual.

Why SCEDs

Single case experimental designs were a mainstay of behavioural studies with animals for many years. In clinical psychology, the health discipline within which SCEDs have the longest tradition, their use arose chiefly from a dissatisfaction both with the shortcomings of the case report described above and an equal dissatisfaction with large-scale randomised controlled trials which, whilst overcoming the problems with cause and effect inherent in case reports, did little to translate group results into statements about what to do with the individual client seen by clinicians in therapeutic situations, particularly when treatment often needed to be individually tailored to client need (Barlow and Hersen, 1984). SCEDs overcome both these problems by combining precise specification of variable with the ability to work with individuals in flexible ways which reflect the needs of clinical practice.

The value of SCEDs

For many clinicians, including one of us (Newell, 1987), SCEDs can represent a first step towards clinical research, because SCEDs contain all the elements of the randomised controlled trial, but can be carried out *during the course of clinical practice*. They thus give us an opportunity for real experiential learning about experimental research, and it is well recognised that such experiential learning is a powerful way of promoting understanding of complex theoretical constructs and practical technologies. Likewise, the SCED can help clinicians seeking to define and develop new interventions. Finally, there are occasions when a particular client difficulty is so unusual that carrying out a group RCT will never represent a practical alternative. Accordingly, the SCED is a powerful learning tool, a useful adjunct to therapeutic innovation and a viable research strategy where no other method of establishing control over variables exists.

SCEDs in clinical practice

It is perhaps surprising that the use of SCEDs in healthcare research has never really taken off, given the flexibility of the approach. healthcare research is characterised by underfunding, and many researchers either combine research with their clinical work or were drawn to research from a need to understand issues in their clinical practice. Yet, the SCED can address both these needs. As a method, the SCED is overwhelmingly intended for use in the context of clinical practice and, as we will see in the following sections, only a short step from the routine measurement of patients' health status which takes place during much clinical practice. As a consequence, it needs result in no additional expense and little, if any additional time input during clinical work. Fascinatingly, it is even possible that SCEDs will decrease time expenditure, because patients will benefit from improved accuracy of assessment and monitoring of their response to treatment. Moreover, because SCEDs are responsive to the changing needs of clients, the method fits well with the patient-centred approach which characterises much healthcare and which has, in the past, led HCPs to be sceptical of what they have perceived to be the mechanistic inflexibility of some quantitative research. Finally, SCEDs will tell the clinician something concrete about whether their interventions are working or not and allow treatments to be adopted and adapted from a position of confidence and expertise. In summary, the HCP using SCEDs to investigate patient problems and the treatment of those problems can do so as part of everyday clinical practice in a way which is individually tailored to each patient and which allows the research process to change alongside the patient's changing needs, whilst retaining the ability to judge cause and effect relationships as they pertain to the treatment approaches being tested (see Deutsch *et al.* [2008] for a recent, simple example of use of a SCED to evaluate an innovative practice in rehabilitation).

Types of SCED

The SCED is a practical approach to controlling the relationship between the independent and dependent variables in the clinical setting. It allows the researcher to attribute cause to the independent variable because it attempts to control intervening variables, through altering the timing at which different levels of the independent variable are introduced. In clinical settings, this typically means the timing of introduction of different treatments and controls (see Chapter 14 for a discussion of these concepts). In the single case experiment, this is done through precise measurement of patient response during the different treatment and control phases. The researcher can draw inferences about whether treatments are affecting patient response by comparing measurements across the different phases. This can be done in two ways. Treatment and control conditions can be introduced and withdrawn sequentially and compared over time (usually, called the AB design or a variant of it) or different treatments can be introduced for different problems with and without withdrawals, and responses to the different problems compared cross-sectionally (the multiple baseline design). These two approaches broadly correspond to the repeated measures and independent groups designs in group studies, respectively (see Chapter 15).

The different types of SCED are designed to deal with threats to internal validity in a number of different ways. The following sections take the clinical example of chronic fatigue and examine how a clinician might use AB and multiple baseline designs to work with a patient to improve their ability to cope with fatigue. The approach taken will look at three well-known approaches to fatigue: energy conservation, exercise and CBT. A detailed description of these approaches is not possible in this chapter, but conservation essentially involves avoiding exertion and doing tasks in as energy efficient a way as possible, whilst exercise exploits the tendency for us to feel less fatigued if our bodies are in better condition. These approaches are offered by a broad range of HCPs (most particularly nurses, physiotherapists and occupational therapists) in different treatment contexts, both formally with people with a diagnosis of chronic fatigue syndrome and with people with chronic fatigue as a concomitant of long-term illnesses. Finally, CBT is a broad pragmatic approach, involving, amongst other things, altering negative thoughts about our problems and ensuring that we give ourselves rewards for carrying out activities and not rewarding ourselves for avoiding activity. In these examples, the effects experienced by the patient are for illustrative purposes only, and should not be taken as an endorsement of any of the treatments concerned.

Measurement and quantification

The first key element of SCED is precise quantification of the person's difficulties and the goals to be attained. In fatigue, it is likely that clinician and patient will agree to rate fatigue and activity using a numerical scale (let us say, a 1–10 scale), as well as goal achievement. Likely goals will include number of hours out of bed, distance walked and ability to concentrate on tasks.

The patient and clinician will agree to use a series of interventions, introducing them one at a time, with baseline measurement in between times, continuing to measure the patient's performance throughout. As well as its usefulness for research, this type of systematic measurement is also therapeutically useful, providing patient and HCP with feedback on the patient's progress (or lack of it).

The AB design

This is the simplest SCED and is defined as the monitoring of behaviour before any intervention is introduced (the A phase), then introducing an intervention (the B phase) at the end of this baseline period, whilst monitoring of performance continues (see Figure 16.1). This design is probably the closest to ordinary clinical practice, and, as a result, is easily used by HCPs as part of their clinical work. However, it contains the major drawback that its ability to allow us to attribute change to the intervention is weak. Although the measurement is systematic, the apparent improvement in subjective fatigue in Figure 16.1 might easily have been caused by some uncontrolled variable (better sleep, better mood) with no relationship to the treatment intervention (conservation).

The most usual way of dealing with this shortcoming is to introduce a return to baseline (the ABA design). In the second A phase, the intervention is withdrawn. In our fatigue example, the patient would be

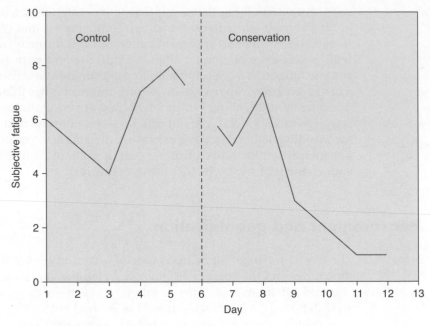

Figure 16.1 The AB design.

asked to stop practicing conservation tactics but to continue to monitor their subjective fatigue (Figure 16.2).

As may be seen, in this example, the increase in fatigue following withdrawal of intervention during the second A phase is taken as evidence of the effectiveness of the intervention. However, for some interventions (e.g. education provision) we would not expect to see a return to baseline, because once something is known, it is not possible to artificially render it unknown again. Accordingly, ABA designs should be assessed in terms of their appropriateness for the treatment being offered. In general, if the treatment requires ongoing input, an ABA design is likely to be appropriate, and will increase our confidence that changes in the dependent variable (fatigue) are a consequence of manipulation of the independent variable (conservation versus no intervention).

The ABAB design

There is also an ethical dilemma with the ABA design, because the patient is left in a situation where, at the end of the study, treatment has been withdrawn. This situation is readily remedied by the reintroduction of the treatment phase, as in the ABAB design (Figure 16.3).

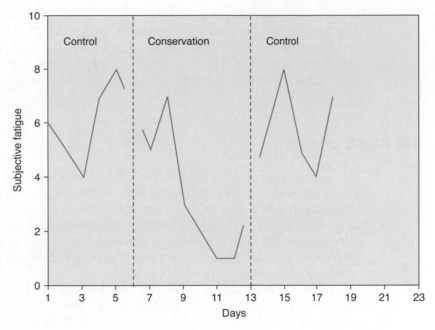

Figure 16.2 The ABA design.

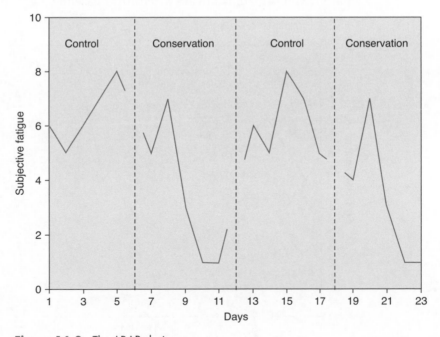

Figure 16.3 The ABAB design.

An additional advantage of this design is that the researcher has further comparison points A1 versus B1, A2 versus B2, A1 versus B2, A1 versus A2. Consistent differences between the A and B points, plus similarity between A1 and A2 would greatly increase our confidence that the independent variable was responsible for changes in the dependent variable.

The ABAC design

In clinical practice, the ABAB approach may be expanded and allow us to introduce a series of different interventions sequentially, each interspersed with a return to baseline. In Figure 16.4, conservation has proved ineffective in reducing fatigue, and so, following a second baseline control (A) phase, a different treatment (exercise) is introduced forming a C phase in the experiment. These are sometimes referred to as ABAC designs. Theoretically, further baseline phases and treatment phases could be added indefinitely, with each treatment phase being designated a different letter – ABACADAEA, and so on.

Notice that this approach reflects the clinical situation where the HCP and client together explore a series of different, potentially effective approaches to the client's difficulties. One important difference is that in SCEDs there is always a return to baseline, permitting better

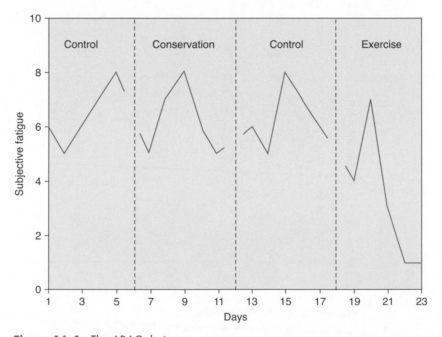

Figure 16.4 The ABAC design.

control of the independent variable. In clinical practice, what most clinicians actually do is omit the baselines (ABCDE). Although this seems to save patient and HCP time, it is not only a weaker research design, because there is only one baseline to measure change against, but potentially *wasteful* of time, because problem assessment will be poorer without good baseline measurement, and the introduction of different treatments may, in consequence, be inappropriate. The ABAC design is extended to include further baseline and a D component featuring, for example, CBT, after both conservation and exercise have been ineffective in altering subjective fatigue (ABACAD).

Where it is acceptable to the patient, we can introduce an element of randomisation, varying both the order in which treatments are introduced and the length of each treatment. This may greatly strengthen our confidence in inferences to be drawn from difference between the treatment and control phases, both by reducing order effects (see Chapter 15) and increasing the range of possible appropriate statistical treatments (Kazdin, 1982). Randomisation also decreases the likelihood that client and therapist are merely capitalising on their observation of naturally occurring fluctuations in behaviour in deciding when to start another phase.

Multiple baseline designs

In AB designs and their variants, we infer cause and effect relationships on the basis of differences between the baseline and treatment phases. The grounds for such inference in multiple baseline designs are slightly different. With such designs, we investigate the effect of interventions on a range of different problems simultaneously, and there is usually no withdrawal of treatment once intervention has begun for each problem. In Figure 16.5, the HCP has used conservation in an effort to increase the range of a patient's activity, exercise to improve their subjective fatigue and CBT to improve their concentration. Although the three approaches have been introduced sequentially, they each address a different problem, all of which have been monitored from the start. Thus, for each problem, there is a different length of monitoring, overlapping with other treatments. In multiple baseline design, the main rationale for inferring cause and effect comes from the comparison of treated and untreated problems *at the same time point*. We infer that treatment is effective by observing differences between patient ratings of the treated and untreated problems. Another approach would be to use the *same* treatment approach for each problem, but to specifically target each problem in turn, whilst maintaining baseline measurement for the untreated ones.

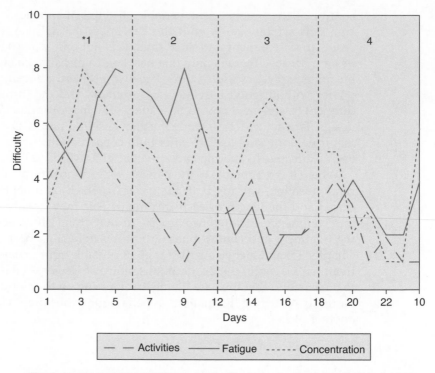

*Time 1 – baseline all conditions; Time 2 – conservation; Time 3 – exercise; Time 4 – cognitive behaviour therapy

Figure 16.5 Multiple baseline designs.

Once again, an element of randomisation can be introduced. Numerous variants on these approaches exist, and the interested reader is directed to Morley (1989) in the first instance.

Data analysis of single case experiments

As might be expected from a method grounded in clinical practice, data analysis has traditionally been simple, usually involving graphing and visual examination of data points as shown in Figures 16.1–16.5 above (see, e.g., Kazdin, 1982). It has been argued that, in clinical practice, complex statistics are not needed, because differences of sufficient size to be important to the patient will be obvious to the observer, and researchers have usually reported on differences between raw scores, mean scores, differences in score levels between the end of one phase and the beginning of another, differences in trend and differences in latency of onset of score changes following a change of phase. However, although visual inspection seems an intuitively valid way of exploring changes in client status which are therapeutically meaningful, there are difficulties with the approach. Important biases appear to operate in the interpretation of visual data (Wampold and Furlong, 1981). Even without such biases, there are compelling reasons to move beyond visual inspection. In clinical settings, the patient is subject to a great number of influences other than treatment, which might interfere with our ability to interpret visual data accurately. Likewise, the baseline data against which changes are judged may be unstable, particularly when there are relatively few data points. Furthermore, if we were involved in developing a new treatment, initial small changes might be indicative of a treatment which, whilst currently weak, showed promise for further development. These might be missed by visual inspection alone.

Finally, small changes are *not* always without importance, particularly if they are repeated or maintained, or increment over time, and therefore result in a level of gain which is useful to the client. This is likely to be particularly the case in interventions which require minimal clinician input. We might be very happy to see small gains as a result of providing simple information, but much less so at the end of a long and expensive period of intensive therapy. These issues are fully described in Kazdin (1982).

Unfortunately, standard statistical tests are rarely suitable for SCEDs, because many of the assumptions of such tests are not adhered to in SCEDs. However, a number of simple statistical alternatives have been developed. These are described briefly in Newell (1992) and fully in Gorman and Allison (1997).

Shortcomings of SCEDs

The level of control available in SCEDs is unlikely ever to approach that of the group experiment, partly because the SCED aims to be responsive to the changing needs of clients during treatment. However, these kinds of difficulties are also present in group designs, including RCTs, and may be avoided or decreased by, for example, manualisation of treatment approaches and systematic replication across many single cases. This latter tactic may also increase confidence in the generalisability of the results of SCEDs. The assumed lack of external validity in SCEDs is also addressed by replication, but advocates of SCEDs have suggested that this is not the only source of enhancing external validity. They suggest that, because human behaviour is lawful (SCEDs were originally developed as part of *radical behaviourism* which sought to identify universal laws of behaviour similar to universal laws of physics and other natural sciences), provided the internal validity of the SCED is appropriate, the findings should hold true in all cases, because they represent demonstrations of universal, generalisable laws of human behaviour. Whilst such universal laws are elusive, our confidence in the findings of an individual SCED will certainly be increased if these findings are in line with theoretical understanding. This, however, is not the same as increased external validity, which, without replication, remains a considerable difficulty for this research method.

HCPs often express ethical concerns about withholding treatment, but baseline recording is important to effective treatment (Kazdin, 1982) because this is part of assessment of the problem, without which treatment would itself be unethical. Likewise, Newell (1992) has suggested that it would only be unethical to withhold a treatment if it were *known* to be effective. If it were not known to be effective, there is no logical ethical offence in withholding it (but see also our comments on this issue in Chapter 5). Moreover, adequate investigation, including baseline measurement, is an important ethical element in offering unproven interventions.

Conclusion

The SCED contains all the main features of large group experiments. Whilst there are obvious disadvantages, such as small numbers, small range of appropriate statistical procedures and poor external validity, there are compelling advantages. The SCED is simple and inexpensive to mount and may be used every day as part of clinical practice. Perhaps the most important consequences of this are that, for patients, their problems are addressed in a way which attempts to assess effectiveness in a structured way and that, for HCPs, they learn about important aspects of experimental design and implementation by direct experience, in a way which would often be impossible using large group studies.

Review questions

What are the main SCED designs?

What is the main difference between ABA designs (and their variants) and multiple baseline designs?

What is the consequence of this difference for how we draw inference about treatment effectiveness from the two types of design?

What are the main arguments for and against statistical analysis in SCEDS?

Exercise

Using Figures 16.1–16.5 as examples, see if you can determine the extent of the changes in between raw scores, differences in score levels between the end of one phase and the beginning of another, differences in trend and differences in latency of onset of changes.

(NB. Because these graphs are for illustration only, there are not enough data points in each phase to calculate mean scores per phase.)

References

Barlow, D.H. and Hersen, M. (1984) *Single Case Experimental Designs*. New York: Pergamon.

Deutsch, J.E., Borbely, M., Filler, J., Huhn, K. and Guarrera-Bowlby, P. (2008) Use of a low-cost, commercially available gaming console (Wii) for rehabilitation of an adolescent with cerebral palsy. *Physical Therapy*, 88(10), 1196–1207.

Gorman, B.S. and Allison, D.B. (1997) Statistical alternatives for single case designs. In: R.D. Franklin, D.B. Allison and B.S. Gorman (eds), *Design and Analysis of Single Case Research*. Mahwah, NJ: Lawrence Erlbaum.

Kazdin, A.E. (1982) *Single Case Research Designs*. New York: Oxford University Press.

Morley, S. (1989) Single case research. In: G. Parry and F.N. Watts (eds), *Behavioural and Mental Health Research: A Handbook of Skills and Methods*. Hove: Lawrence Erlbaum.

Newell, R.J. (1987) Treatment of irritable bowel syndrome by exposure in fantasy: a case report. *Behavioural Psychotherapy*, 15, 381–387.

Newell, R.J. (1992) The single case experiment: a research method for everyday use. *Nursing Practice*, 6(1), 24–27.

Wampold, B.E. and Furlong, M.J. (1981) The heuristics of visual inspection. *Behavioral Assessment*, 3, 79–92.

Further reading

Busk, P.L. and Marascuilo, L.A. (1992) Statistical analysis in single-case research: issues, procedures and recommendations with applications to multiple behaviors. In: T.R. Kratchowill and J.R. Levin (eds), *Single Case Research and Analysis*. Hillsdale, NJ: Lawrence Erlbaum.

Kratchowill, T.R. and Levin, J.R. (eds) (1992) *Single Case Research and Analysis*. Hillsdale, NJ: Lawrence Erlbaum.

Randomised Controlled Trials

Key points

- A randomised controlled trial (RCT) is a type of experiment.
- RCTs involve randomisation, a control group and manipulation of the independent variable.
- RCTs attempt to control bias.
- RCTs are the most effective way of examining cause and effect relationships, including the effect of treatment on patients.
- Explanatory trials possess high internal validity and establish what principle, mechanism or theory accounts for a change in patient condition.
- Pragmatic trials possess high external validity and establish how well a principle, mechanism or theory translates into the real clinical world.
- RCTs are essential in providing patients with accurate information about therapeutic interventions.

Introduction

In healthcare, the randomised controlled trial (RCT), first adopted in medicine, has come to be regarded as the gold standard in investigating

Research for Evidence-Based Practice in Healthcare, Second edition, by Robert Newell and Philip Burnard
© 2011 Robert Newell and Philip Burnard

treatment effectiveness. Its use has spread from simple medical and surgical interventions to embrace nursing, allied health professions and social care, and the investigation of complex multi-method healthcare interventions and aspects of service delivery. There are two reasons for this increased use of RCTs. First, in healthcare, it is important for us to have a clear idea about whether treatments we offer are effective. To do this, we need to be equally clear that something other than the treatment we are investigating is not, in fact, causing any improvement in the patient's health status. If we cannot be clear about these two things, we have no justification in offering the treatment to patients. Second, RCTs are currently the best way of achieving that clarity, because no other research method is as good at controlling for these possible alternative sources of patient improvement. In this chapter, we will explore what RCTs are, how they go about establishing whether or not an intervention works, the issues which researchers need to consider in using RCT methodology and the practicalities of designing and undertaking RCTs.

What is an RCT?

An RCT is a special kind of experiment which investigates the effectiveness of therapeutic interventions with patients. To understand this further, we need to know a little about the nature of experiments, which we examined in detail in Chapter 15. Essentially, experiments attempt to explore whether there are cause and effect relationships between particular events in the world and are regarded as doing a good job of this because they are good at controlling bias. The RCT brings together the elements of experimental research in the context of healthcare research; because the RCT is so central to healthcare research, many of the issues of experimentation discussed earlier are revisited in the current chapter.

As we saw in Chapter 15, bias is controlled by manipulating the independent variable (the thing we think may be causing some effect in the world) between two or more groups and seeing whether this manipulation has an effect on the dependent variable (the thing we think might be being affected). At the same time, bias is further controlled by trying to remove from the picture unwanted intervening or confounding variables which might interfere with our ability to attribute changes in the dependent variable to our manipulation of the independent variable.

In RCTs, the independent variable is some form of health intervention which is varied by the researcher over two or more conditions. Condition here does not mean an illness or health problem. This is simply an unfortunate jargon carry over from experimental method in general and loosely means group. Thus, if we speak of a treatment condition, we mean a treatment group – those people receiving a particular intervention. Now, in an RCT, the intervention is consciously applied to one group of participants (usually, patients) rather than another. This is what is meant by manipulation. It differs from simply observing naturally occurring variations, because we *decide* what the variation is to be, *define* it in precise terms and *apply* it to one group rather than another.

One alternative to manipulation would be to observe naturally occurring variations. We might, for example, look at patients from two different wards where two different models of care were in use and compare the two groups. However, this would be less useful than the manipulation of such models of care between different groups because of the increased potential for bias. The two wards might differ in all sorts of ways which had nothing to do with the model of care employed. For example, all the staff on one of the ward might be more experienced than those on another, or the patient groups might be different in terms of the complaints from which they suffered, their age, sex, or whatever.

These are very obvious differences, and easy to spot, but many such differences are more subtle. Let us say we worked in a setting where a multidisciplinary care pathway was to be introduced sequentially onto two different wards (Wards 1 and 2) with similar staff groups, both of which dealt with identical patients. We wanted to see whether the care pathway had any effect on patient improvement and decided to compare the two wards. It seems as if two major sources of unwanted difference between the wards have been sorted out. However, suppose that, unknown to us, the person responsible for introducing the pathway had chosen to introduce it onto Ward 1 rather than Ward 2 because the staff on Ward 1 were more enthusiastic and open to change. Clearly, their enthusiasm would be a powerful potential confounding variable, and might be just as much the source of any difference between the wards as the care pathway.

This, then, is the first requirement of an RCT – deliberate, conscious manipulation of the independent variable, rather than observation of naturally occurring variability. By contrast with observation, manipulation allows us to control bias by reducing the likelihood that some other difference between the two conditions, rather than the difference between the conditions we claimed was responsible, might be causing any observed differences in response between the conditions. When we manipulate the variable to be studied, we do so precisely in order to isolate, as far as possible, the entity we believe might be responsible for changes in patient status. This factor – the ability to isolate the independent variable from the effects of unwanted variables – is the sole factor which drives the act of manipulation.

Manipulation rather than observation also allows us to stipulate precisely what the independent variable will consist of. So, in the care pathway example, we can develop precise definitions of what constitutes the pathway, what the health professionals concerned will be required to do as part of implementing it and what training they will require in order for us to be confident they are implementing it adequately. At the same time, we can specify what care patients who are not receiving the pathway will receive, and part of that specification will involve ensuring that their care truly is different from that involved in the care pathway. This process is often referred to as specifying, defining or operationalising the independent variable, but all these terms mean the same thing – stipulating exactly what the manipulation will consist of and ensuring that such a manipulation will take place.

Often, the goals of excluding confounding variables and adequately operationalising the independent variable are very hard to achieve, but as a general rule, a manipulated variable (as in an RCT or other experiment) offers far greater possibility for precise definition than a variable in an observational study.

The second element of the RCT is the notion of randomness of the manipulation of the independent variable (intervention) between groups involved. This is closely linked to the idea of manipulation, because it is a way of avoiding the problem we encountered above – the possibility that uncontrolled variables might be responsible for differences between the groups. In the above example, this problem involved selection bias – our HCPs were chosen on the basis of enthusiasm, which might have affected patients. A similar thing might happen if we offered treatment to patients on a first-come, first-served basis, with first-comers receiving the experimental treatment. Unfortunately, first-comers might differ from others in all sorts of ways other than the treatment they go on to receive (more motivated, more affluent, more sick, more desperate, to name just a few). Similar problems arise in almost any kind of non-random sample, because we cannot be confident that members of the two groups are similar, and this kind of subject variability can considerably affect our results.

In the RCT, confounding variables arising from selection difficulties are typically avoided by means of random allocation to treatment or control groups. In all cases, the principal reason for randomisation is to ensure that each member of the entire group of participants has a fair chance of being allocated to either the experimental or control group, and the reason for wanting this fair chance is to ensure that possible differences between individual participants are roughly equally distributed between the groups. Randomisation does not *guarantee* that this will be the case, but is a necessary minimum safeguard against the possible confounding effects of subject variability.

However, even the act of randomisation is prone to potential bias, and, as a result, specific protocols for randomisation exist. Traditional methods of randomisation, such as the use of putting cards bearing allocations to the different conditions into sealed envelopes have been found to be subject to abuse, as the people carrying out the randomisation have sought to influence allocation (e.g., by holding the envelope to the light in order to see its contents without opening). Partly, in consequence, the gold standard for randomisation is via remote, telephone randomisation using computer-generated allocation and performed by someone unconnected with the clinical work and the conduct of the rest of the study. This approach is resilient to abuse, as far as we know.

The final important feature of RCTs is the ability to assign participants to a *control group*. In experiments, usually only one group receives the experimental procedure, whilst the other receives some procedure which is in all respects similar to the experimental one, but lacks the novel element. However, in complex studies, there may be many novel treatments in a single study. Each treatment will be clearly defined and offered to one group only, so that there will be no overlap between the treatments received by each group. Finally, there will be a group of individuals who receive some intervention which is *not* novel. These are the control group and are the standard against which the novel treatments are judged. Typically, the most important question in an RCT is whether or not there is a difference between the novel treatment (experimental group) and the control treatment (control group). In a well-conducted RCT, the experimental and control groups will vary only by virtue of the fact that they receive differing treatments. These different treatments will be so well specified that they represent some single, clear difference in treatment.

Confusingly, the control treatment may, in fact, be no treatment at all, although this is generally regarded as the weakest form of control. This is because no treatment controls in RCTs do little to account for non-specific effects of treatment or from unwanted effects of experiments in general. For example, it is well known in psychotherapy that such issues as the personality, social skills, enthusiasm of a therapist can exert some therapeutic influence. In healthcare and medicine, the communication skills of the clinician can affect compliance with therapeutic regimes and, therefore, indirectly, the effectiveness of such regimes. More broadly, in research as a whole, the effect of attention on research subjects is itself known to influence their responses. In no-treatment control RCTs, it is often impossible to tease out non-specific effects such as attention, from the effects of the independent variable.

One of the commonest tactics, in assigning patients to a control group, has been the use of a waiting list control. This is simply one example of a no-treatment control group, but is particularly weak, because not only are the control group receiving none of the non-specific effects of being in any treatment, but they are also *expecting* to receive treatment in the future, which may give rise to any number of thoughts, feelings and behaviours which would affect their scores and erroneously lead us to believe that differences between them and people in the experimental group arose from specific effects of the novel treatment. However, on the plus side, it must be noted that no-treatment controls are immeasurably better than no controls at all! Moreover, there are many situations where no-treatment controls of one kind or another are the only practical solution.

Sometimes, it is possible to introduce some form of *attention control*, which attempts to offer participants all the non-specific aspects of treatment without the specific component under investigation *and* give participants the same amount of attention (e.g., through the interviewing and the assessment process) as they would receive in active treatment. There are two problems with this tactic. The first is an ethical one, in that the researcher will not wish to waste participants' time by offering what are essentially 'filler' treatments – activities which fill time in an apparently meaningful way which has no demonstrable benefit. The second problem is purely practical. Even if it were ethical to offer patients non-specific interventions to control for the non-specific and attention effects of a particular novel treatment, we might run into difficulties finding a non-specific intervention which was convincing to patients. Administering an unconvincing 'filler' treatment might have quite the reverse effect from our intention of offsetting non-specific therapeutic effects as it would give rise to non-specific *negative* effects in the control group.

In a great deal of healthcare research, but also in much health service research which examines complex healthcare interventions, a tradition has arisen of using best current available treatment as the control intervention. There are considerable advantages to this. By and large, the best current available treatment will be what the patient is currently receiving, although this may vary from place to place. It will be a credible alternative, both to patients and clinicians. It will contain broadly the same non-specific aspects as the novel treatment. Finally, it will represent a 'gold standard' against which to judge the novel treatment.

Explanatory versus pragmatic trials

In Chapter 13, we examined internal validity (essentially the amount of confidence we can have that changes in the dependent variable are caused by the action of the independent or that lack of such changes are caused by lack of action of the independent variable) and external validity (basically, the likelihood that things we have observed in an experiment are likely to be transferable to similar situations away from the experimental environment).

There is always a tension between these two components of validity in experiments. Increasing the internal validity of a study inevitably means decreasing its external validity and vice versa. Let us illustrate this point by returning to the example of the care pathway. We will want to be certain that patients on the pathway truly receive care in line with the care pathway, and will take certain measures to ensure we can assert this. For example, we will ensure proper training in the use of the pathway for all staff, and perhaps give them a brief examination to ensure the training has been effective. This is known as a manipulation check and is a design strength. We will also ensure that the patients on the pathway are only cared for by doctors, nurses, healthcare assistants, physiotherapists and occupational therapists who have undergone this training. All this is fine and is an important factor in establishing the internal validity of the RCT, because it increases our confidence that differences between pathway and non-pathway patients are truly caused by the presence of the pathway. However, the sceptic can easily argue that our RCT lacks external validity because it does not represent how *real* care pathways are practiced in the clinical world. In this world, they may argue, training is imperfect and healthcare workers swap between different care settings, they also forget what they have learnt and are not being constantly primed to remember it by being given tests of knowledge. They would further argue that, to be important, a care pathway should be sufficiently robust to withstand these interferences.

So, which view is right? The answer, as with so many aspects of clinical research, is that both are. We want certainty that it truly is the treatment that is causing changes in patient well-being (so far as anyone can have such certainty) and it is the presence of internal validity which allows this certainty. But we also want a treatment which is valuable to patients *in general*, not just to that small subgroup who take part in the artificial setting of RCTs. We need high external validity to ensure that. Accordingly, RCTs are generally divided into *explanatory trials*, which aim to identify some underlying principle of treatment, and *pragmatic trials*, which aim to investigate that principle in the real world of everyday practice and see if it still applies there. In our pathway example, an explanatory trial would try to do at least the following:

Explanatory RCT of multidisciplinary care pathway

Isolate the key elements of a pathway

Incorporate these into the experimental condition of the study

Ensure the control condition did not contain any of them

Ensure adequate training of staff in the experimental condition in using the pathway

Monitor use of the pathway throughout the trial

Control non-pathway elements of care (e.g. patients' consultant) across the conditions

Control non-pathway characteristics of staff (e.g. age, qualifications, experience) across conditions

Control patient characteristics (age; severity of complaint)

In brief, as much control as possible over likely confounding variables would be exercised, in order to give a picture of something as close to a pure delivery of the pathway as is feasible. The reason for this is because we want to know whether the key elements of a pathway (the things which make it a pathway and which exemplify the theory or rationale behind constructing a pathway) affect patient care. In other words, we attempt to *explain* what (if anything) it is about pathways which makes a difference. Explanatory trials are very important in the early stages of developing or testing a new treatment, because they enable us to isolate the active ingredients, and also because, as they are so good at controlling unwanted variables, they increase the likelihood that differences between the treatment and control groups will be detected, because these differences are less likely to be swamped by the action of uncontrolled variables.

The pragmatic trial is then undertaken as an important next step. Whilst the steps described above to ensure that the experimental and control groups are truly different are still important, there are other considerations in pragmatic trials which interact with these. In a pragmatic trial, we will want to:

Pragmatic RCT of multidisciplinary care pathway

Ensure that the treatment can be delivered by a clinicians across a broad range of experience, age, qualification

Ensure that the training given is practicable in ordinary clinical settings

Allow variability of patient characteristics

Allow variability of non-pathway elements of treatment (such as consultant procedure preferences)

Essentially, what these different concerns in a pragmatic trial are trying to do is ensure that our treatment is sufficiently robust to stand up to the many uncontrolled sources of variation in patient response which happen in the real world. It is often suggested that explanatory trials are at the research end of R&D whilst pragmatic trials are closer to the development end, but both use the same general principles of experimental design.

In many ways, the tension between and different rationales for these two sorts of RCT encapsulate the whole point of undertaking RCTs at all. RCTs are often criticised for not capturing the entirety of complex interventions in healthcare. There is no doubt that this is so, but the criticism misses the point. Proponents of RCTs do not, generally, wish to capture such complexity, and, indeed many will claim that this is impossible to do, either using RCTs or any other methodological approaches.

Rather, people who undertake RCTs are principally interested in answering the question: What is the necessary and sufficient intervention to make a difference which the patient desires? Clearly, we want our intervention to be sufficient, because if it were not, we would not be helping patients to achieve the changes they wanted. Proponents of RCTs argue that the robust control of bias is the best chance we have of being able confidently to tell patients that a given intervention is effective (sufficient) for their difficulties. However, we also want the treatment to be necessary, as the inclusion of unnecessary elements would be a waste of patient time and energy and, therefore, unethical. This provides one rationale for seeking to isolate particular elements of treatment responsible for patient improvement. The other motivation for so doing is that isolating these active therapeutic components means that we may be also able to apply them in similar situations, rather than starting from scratch, because we know which specific component of an intervention is causing the change and we know the principle behind its action.

RCTs are often thought to be the special preserve of medical practitioners, and this has in itself led to opposition from other healthcare professionals, whether because they wish to establish professional and methodological distance from their medical colleagues or because they perceive RCT as being associated with a mechanistic approach to treatment. However, these views are difficult to support. In my own work (RN), for example, I have explored with both medical and non-medical colleagues issues as diverse as the impact of self-help materials on disfigurement (Newell and Clarke, 2000), the feasibility of using entonox in bone marrow biopsy (Johnson *et al.*, 2008), the contribution made by advocacy to access to services in learning disability (Raghavan *et al.*, 2009). All these pieces of research were nurse-led RCTs. More importantly, however, these studies could equally well and have been led by *any* member of the multidisciplinary team. Indeed, pragmatic RCTs are now a standard approach in non-medically driven healthcare.

Just a few examples will serve to show the breadth of what can be achieved by RCTs in healthcare, other than the traditional use of RCTs to compare two drugs or other medical treatments. For example, a complex rehabilitation intervention following stroke and hip fracture was examined by Ryan *et al.* (2006) using a single blind RCT. In a more traditional use of RCT methodology, Langley *et al.* (2006) compared aspects of recovery after second-degree tears in labour following suturing or non-suturing of the tear, whilst Clifford *et al.* (2002) examined different approaches to community medications monitoring. In the field of radiography, Bartholomew and colleagues compared two different methods of undertaking computerised skull X-rays, demonstrating, incidentally, that the use of RCTs is by no means confined to comparisons between *treatments*. In this case, the comparative merits of two approaches to an *investigative* procedure were examined. It is also worth noting that all the examples of RCTs given here were undertaken either by, or in close collaboration with, people involved in day-to-day clinical practice.

Finally, pragmatic trials increase our ability to be able to confidently tell a patient that this intervention we have worked long and hard to develop and test is likely to work for them in routine clinical practice, as opposed being effective only in the rarified world of the RCT. Taken as a whole, RCTs, whilst often difficult to design in clinical practice, represent the most robust test of cause and effect. In consequence, the evidence derived from them is essential to practice and the appropriate communication of that practice to patients. Without RCTs, it would be difficult to give patients accurate information, and without *that* they would be unable to make informed choices about treatment.

Review questions

What are the necessary components of an RCT?
What do they aim to do?
What are the different aims of explanatory and pragmatic RCTs?
What are the implications of these aims for how the two types of trial are conducted?

Exercise

The distinction between explanatory and pragmatic trials is not always as clear cut as we have suggested here. Often, practical considerations determine some of the choices made about internal and external validity.

Identify an RCT relevant to your clinical practice and ask the following questions:

How far is this study a pragmatic or explanatory trial?
How good is the internal validity and why?
How good is the external validity and why?

References

Clifford, R.M., Batty, K.T., Davis, T.M.E., Davis, W., Stein, G., Stewart, G. and Plumridge, R. (2002) A randomised controlled trial of a pharmaceutical care programme in high-risk diabetic patients in an outpatient clinic. *International Journal of Pharmacy Practice*, 10, 85–90.

Johnson, H., Burke, J., Newell, R., Plews, C. and Priapia, L. (2008) Improving the patient's experience of a bone marrow biopsy. Nitrous oxide analgesia vs placebo in bone marrow biopsy: a double blind randomised controlled trial. *Journal of Clinical Nursing*, 17(6), 717–725.

Langley, V., Thoburn, A., Shaw, S. and Barton, A. (2006) Second degree tears: to suture or not? A randomized controlled trial. *British Journal of Midwifery*, 14(9), 550–554.

Newell, R. and Clarke, M. (2000) Evaluation of a self-help leaflet in treatment of social difficulties following facial disfigurement. *International Journal of Nursing Studies*, 37, 381–388.

Raghavan, R., Wassem, F., Newell, R. and Small, N. (2009) A randomised controlled trial of liaison worker model for young people with learning disabilities and mental health problems. *Journal of Applied Research in Intellectual Disabilities*, 22, 256–263.

Ryan, T., Enderby, P. and Rigby, A.S. (2006) A randomized controlled trial to evaluate intensity of community-based rehabilitation provision following stroke or hip fracture in old age. *Clinical Rehabilitation*, 20(2), 123–131.

Further reading

Bartholomew, A.L., Denton, E.R.E., Shaw, M. and Marshall, T.J. (2004) A randomised controlled trial comparing lateral skull computerised radiographs with or without a grid. *Radiography*, 10(3), 201–204.

Getliffe, K. (1998) Developing a protocol for a randomised controlled trial: factors to consider. *Nurse Researcher*, 6(1), 5–17.

Polit, D.F., Beck, C.T. and Hungler, B.P. (2001) *Essentials of Nursing Research: Methods, Appraisal and Utilization*. Philadelphia: Lippincott.

Sibbald, B. and Roland, M. (1998) Why are randomised controlled trials important? *British Medical Journal*, 316, 201.

Watson, B., Proctor, S. and Cochrane, W. (2004) Using randomised controlled trials (RCTs) to test service interventions: issues of standardisation, selection and generalisability. *Nurse Researcher*, 11(3), 28–42.

Website

http://www.phru.nhs.uk/Doc_Links/rct%20appraisal%20tool.pdf

Non-Experimental Approaches

Key points

- Non-experimental approaches involve observation of naturally occurring relationships and differences between variables.
- Non-experimental approaches are useful when experimental approaches are unethical or impractical.
- Causal inference is weak in non-experimental approaches.
- Descriptive designs only describe relationships between variables.
- Causal-comparative designs (comparative/ex post facto designs) compare two or more naturally occurring groups.
- Correlational designs explore relationships between variables in a single group.
- Some correlational approaches allow prediction through the assignment of predictor variables.

Introduction

In various ways, all four previous chapters have been concerned with the specification and manipulation of variables. The amount of time

Research for Evidence-Based Practice in Healthcare, Second edition, by Robert Newell and Philip Burnard
© 2011 Robert Newell and Philip Burnard

we have devoted to these notions partly reflects the need for precision in understanding both the practicalities of conducting experiments and partly the importance of this type of approach in providing a robust rationale for employing one healthcare intervention rather than another. However, there are many times when experimental and quasi-experimental approaches are inappropriate.

At an early stage in the life of a research question, it is often difficult to frame hypotheses with regard to the cause and effect, and often difficult to specify what interventions might prove potentially useful for patient difficulties. At this stage, experimentation is unlikely to help us, and we are more likely to want to describe the issues under debate. There are also times when there are ethical problems with experimental approaches. It may, for example, be felt that withholding treatment from patients is unwise or unfair, and so we may want to examine naturally occurring differences between groups by, for example, examining the treatments given for a particular patient difficulty in different hospitals or units. Finally, there may be times when the use of an experimental approach is simply impractical, because, for example, we want to observe the relationship between different aspects of people's behaviour or environment.

In these three situations, non-experimental quantitative approaches are probably the best available alternative, and can greatly assist us in understanding more about the problem under review. Non-experimental research differs from experimental and quasi-experimental research in the important sense that no manipulation of the independent variable occurs (although naturally occurring variation in that variable may be observed). Indeed, in the three examples we gave in the previous paragraph, we have actually outlined the three main types of non-experimental quantitative research: descriptive research, causal-comparative and correlational. As the names suggest, these three designs aim to describe phenomena, compare naturally occurring groups and examine the correlation (relatedness) of characteristics in naturally occurring groups. One important warning here is that the causal-comparative approach suffers from a certain imprecision of language, because by definition, non-experimental approaches cannot determine cause and effect. Finally, some commentators have suggested that correlational and causal-comparative designs are really just subtypes of descriptive research, because the only meaningful distinction is between manipulation and observation (that is to say, between experimental and quasi-experimental research on the one hand, and descriptive research on the other).

Although, the implication that such a cause–effect relationship exists may be very strong in certain cases, it still requires formal testing in an experimental approach to give us adequate confidence that such a relationship exists. This is because without the checks and balances of an experimental design, we can never be certain that some variable we have not suspected or have been unable to control for has not led to the observed relationship between the variables in a non-experimental study. We shall give some examples of why this might be so when we look at causal-comparative and correlational design below, but it is also well worth your reviewing the discussions of this topic in the previous four chapters.

Descriptive designs

In this type of design, the level of causal inference possible is lowest. However, this is not a drawback, because the intention of such designs is not to establish cause–effect relationships (or should not be!). These designs simply allow us to describe the nature of the phenomenon of interest to us. Typically, this is done using descriptive statistics to report frequencies, means, ranges and so on (see Chapter 20). Methods for descriptive research are essentially observational. This observation may involve the following.

Observational research

- Observation in real life (noting the number of times nurses wash their hands on a shift of duty, the duration of washing on each occasion, the type of washing agent used on each occasion, the types of procedure performed before washing occurs).
- Scrutiny of existing records (number of patients with multiple sclerosis seen in a neurology clinic; number referred to occupational therapist, number presenting with different difficulties [pain, fatigue], advice offered by the therapist).
- Specifically designed survey (patient description of the occurrence of psychosocial difficulties following prostatectomy).

These three broad approaches basically underlie almost all descriptive research. For example, large epidemiological studies are essentially either done by scrutiny of existing records, survey or a combination of both. Descriptive approaches can follow up people over an extended period of time (cohort studies, longitudinal studies), or take a snapshot of them on a single occasion (cross-sectional studies). The ingredient which underlies all quantitative descriptive work is the use of large samples and the use of descriptive statistics to organise the resulting large data sets in a way which is meaningful to the consumer of research. By contrast, qualitative descriptive and observational studies typically examine the views and experiences of small numbers in depth.

Causal comparative designs (comparative designs/ex post facto designs)

We touched in passing on the comparative approach in Chapter 16, when we pointed out that comparing the responses of men and women was not really experimental because no manipulation of the independent variable took place. As we noted, you cannot (yet!) randomly assign living people to one gender or another. You can, however, observe ways in which their responses vary. For example, if we gave men and women with chronic fatigue the standard intervention (cognitive behaviour therapy) and observed their differing response to treatment, we might well conclude that women did better than men. We might also want to conclude that this was *because* of their being men or women. In other words, we would want to assert a relationship between the supposed independent variable (gender) and the supposed dependent variable (response to treatment). You will notice that we have put in the word 'supposed' here. This is because the language of independent and dependent variables is associated with experimental method and is, therefore, an implicit assertion of causation. It is perfectly proper to regard gender here as *acting in the role of the independent variable*, but it is important to note that the degree of causal attribution advisable in the causal-comparative approach is far smaller than in experimental and quasi-experimental approaches. This is because, once again, without manipulation, we cannot be sure that the action of the independent variable has caused changes in the independent variable. For example, suppose we compare the school achievements of children who have been involved in after-school clubs with those who have not. We find that club attenders have a higher achievement than non-attenders. We want to assert that after-school clubs improve achievement, but is it fair to do so? The parents of club attenders might be more motivated towards education, and so might be providing their children with more educational stimulation in the home. Equally, they might be working long hours in well-paid jobs and so need the extra supervision time an after-school club provides, but might be using their extra income to enrich their children's education in a number of ways. In non-experimental comparative research, we have limited opportunities to control for possible intervening variables of this kind, and in the example just given, a true experimental approach, if possible, would have been a much stronger design. Nevertheless, the causal-comparative approach is invaluable for situations where manipulation of the independent variable is impossible. It is essentially similar to an experiment, but without the element of manipulation. Typically, it is used in situations where participants are already a member of one group or another (e.g. men versus women, nurses versus physiotherapists, inpatients versus outpatients) hence the alternative title of ex post facto (after the fact) designs. Finally, some commentators reserve the expression 'causal-comparative' for studies which combine elements of comparative and correlational designs.

A causal comparative study

Causal comparative design in a survey of attitudes to medication
  In the large study cited below, the researchers asked doctors and pharmacists about their views on different medication formulations for people with diabetes. They then compared the responses of doctors and pharmacists.
  Baqir, W. and Maguire, A. (2001) Doctors' and pharmacists' attitudes to the use of sugar-free and sugar-containing medicines in the elderly. *International Journal of Pharmacy Practice*, 9, 177–184.

Case–control studies

In the case–control approach, the researcher decides on a particular attribute (e.g. an illness, outcome or ability), then divides a group of individuals into those who do and do not have that attribute. The researcher then asks what other characteristics these individuals have and sees whether those in the two groups differ in the extent to which they possess these other characteristics. Many of you may know that early studies of the impact of smoking on lung cancer were case–control studies. Thus, the researchers looked at a group of people with and without lung cancer and asked what other characteristics they possessed. The key difference between the two groups was that those with cancer were smokers. We are not, however, restricted to the investigation of illness. For example, we might want to know what factors influence attendance at routine breast screening appointments. One way would be to look at women who did and did not attend such appointments and see what characteristics distinguished between them. In this context, those who attended would be the 'cases'. From examining the medical records of all women who had been invited to attend, we might see patterns related to (for instance) age, social class, educational attendance, previous patterns of GP attendance, postcode, distance from the screening centre. Using statistical methods, we could see which of these factors differed significantly between the groups, and even combine the factors together, to see if they influenced one another in the ways that they differed between groups. As you can perhaps see, the case–control design is one particular variant of the causal comparative approach, because it compares people according to unmanipulated membership of one group or another, which the researcher observes and uses as the basis for comparison. In common with other causal comparative approaches, the case–control approach is weakened by lack of randomisation or other manipulation of an independent variable.

Case–control study

Case–control study of consequences of mobile phone use

Use of mobile phones has been suggested to lead to brain tumours. This well-conducted multidisciplinary case–control study from Japan found no increased risk of glioma or meningioma.

Takebayashi, T., Varsier, N., Kikuchi, Y., Wake, W., Taki, M., Watanabe, S., Akiba, S. and amaguchi, N. (2008) Mobile phone use, exposure to radiofrequency electromagnetic field, and brain tumour: a case–control study. *British Journal of Cancer*, 98, 652–659.

Cohort studies

While the case–control study begins with the index attribute (lung cancer, attendance at screening) and investigates possible causative factors, the cohort study starts with a group of people who have the possibility of exposure to possible causative factors and looks at the relationship between exposure to the factors and eventual outcomes. As with case–control studies, cohort studies are most often seen in the field of epidemiology, and so are most often described in terms of exposure to risk factors for disease and the eventual rates of development of the disease by those who have different levels of exposure to these risks. However, we can once again consider its use in a broader context. For example, in an investigation of attempts to reduce teenage pregnancy, we might follow up all young teenage girls over 5 years and compare those who had and had not been offered contraceptive advice in school, looking at the pregnancy rates in the two groups over time. Here, we are asserting that exposure to the supposed causative factor (contraceptive advice) results in an increased risk of *not* becoming pregnant.

Although, in the example we have just given, the cohort in the study is examined for one specific risk factor (advice) related to one particular outcome, a cohort could be examined for many different risk factors related to many outcomes. In each case, the group would be divided into those exposed or not exposed to the risk said to relate to the particular outcome. This is particularly likely to occur in large cohorts such as birth cohorts.

Use of a birth cohort to examine cardiac risk factors

Cohort study of cardiac risk factors

This recent public health study shows the potential for large cohorts to continue to yield valuable healthcare results over an extended period of time.

Cooper, R., Atherton, K. and Power, C. (2009) Gestational age and risk factors for cardiovascular disease: evidence from the 1958 British birth cohort followed to mid-life. *International Journal of Epidemiology*, 38, 235–244.

Correlational designs

Unlike comparative designs, correlational designs do not rely on participants being in two or more groups in order to examine differences between them. By contrast, in correlational research we are interested in how two different variables relate to each other in any member of a group. For example, we might be interested in the relationship between smoking and alcohol intake. Naturally, we cannot artificially induce one group of people to smoke whilst allowing others to abstain. We can, however, observe what happens to people's smoking behaviour as their alcohol intake rises, either on particular occasions or with regard to their intake over extended periods. We can then see whether there is any systematic relationship between the two variables (e.g. number of cigarettes smoked and blood alcohol levels [over a short period] or number of cigarettes reported smoked and number of units of alcohol drunk [over an extended period]).

Correlations can be positive (as scores on one variable rise so do scores on the other) or negative (as scores on one variable increase, scores on the other decrease). Levels of correlation vary between 0.0 (no relationship at all) and 1.0 (perfect positive correlation) or −1.0 (perfect negative correlation). Deciding what constitutes a strong or weak correlation is not an exact science, but generally a score of 1.0 to 0.7 would be regarded as strong, <0.7 to 0.3 as moderate to weak and <0.3 as weak to none for positive correlations. Different writers apply different criteria, and it is worth recognising that different cut-offs might be appropriate in different circumstances. For example, in exploratory work, we might not want to write off even correlations lower than 0.3. It is also possible to conduct multiple correlations to assess the relationships between many different variables as they interact with each other in the environment. In the example above, we might, for example, follow up people over time with regard to their calorific intake and frequency of exercise, as well as the cigarette and nicotine consumption, giving us a more rounded picture of their health-related behaviours. We could then examine the individual correlations between each pair of variables, but also the relationship of each with the other three.

Characteristics of correlations

Correlations can be

positive (as one variable increases, so does the other, as one variable decreases, so does the other)
negative (as one variable increases, the other decreases)
linear or non-linear
strong, moderate or weak

All the above discussion is based on the idea that correlations are *linear*. That is to say, one variable rises by the same amount (or by a multiple of the same amount) as the other in a simple positive correlation between two variables (see Figure 18.1).

However, sometimes this kind of relationship does not exist. For example, it might be the case that, in the smoking example, alcohol intake and smoking intake rise together for some people, but not for others. Some of these participants might, for example, show a pattern

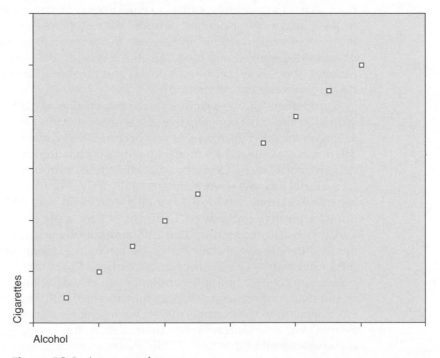

Figure 18.1 Linear correlation.

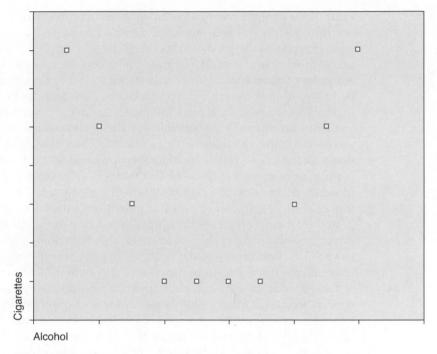

Figure 18.2 Non-linear correlation.

where smoking is relatively constant, whilst alcohol patterns are variable, whilst for others, alcohol and smoking show a negative correlation. In Figure 18.2, participants near the left side of the graph show this negative correlation, those in the middle of the graph show a constant rate of smoking regardless of alcohol intake, whilst those at the right show a positive correlation. As you might imagine, it is often difficult to spot non-linear correlations or to interpret their importance. Moreover, simply running a statistical test would not reveal this pattern of interaction – you have to see it graphically displayed.

Correlation and prediction

One of the interesting (and potentially powerful) features of correlational designs is that it is possible to move beyond describing the relationship between variables towards the modelling of the comparative *impact* of different variables on others, often in complex interactions. In these situations, researchers use statistical techniques to specify one or more of the variables as *predictor* variables, which essentially involves assigning to such variables the role of an independent variable which can be used to predict responses on the other variables. The assignment of predictor variables can be changed around to see which ones best account for the changes in the others. Again, returning to our earlier example, we might regard alcohol intake as the predictor variable and see how well it predicts smoking, diet and exercise, or we might regard exercise as the predictor and see how well it predicts alcohol intake, smoking and diet. Two things should be stressed here. First, our assignment of one variable as a predictor variable once again tempts us to regard it as causal, but in correlational research, as in other non-experimental research, there is always the danger that unconsidered variables are actually responsible for the relationships we think we see between the variables being examined. Thus, our degree of confidence in the causal link is considerably lowered. Second, sometimes it is possible to appeal to theoretical constructs or to other aspects of the research design (e.g. the care with which participants have been chosen, or the unlikelihood of causal explanations other than the one suggested by the observed relationships) to increase our confidence in the integrity of the causal chain. However, the assertions of causality on the basis of non-experimental research require sensitivity and experience and are never free from the possibility of alternative explanations.

One special case of non-experimental research is the survey. It is special because it often yields large amounts of observational descriptive data which can be combined by the researcher in many different ways to give rise to a whole range of tests, some of which represented comparative designs whilst others reflect a correlational approach, all within the same study. The practicalities of survey research are examined in the next chapter.

Review questions

What differentiates experimental from non-experimental research?
Why might we want to do non-experimental, rather than experimental research?
What differentiates causal-comparative from correlational research?

Exercise

Look again at the example of nurse handwashing. We gave it as an example of descriptive research, but you could extend it using comparative and correlational approaches to explore differences and relationships in the study situation. How would you go about doing this? What variables would you look at? Which are comparative? Which are correlational? What if you were to compare frequency of handwashing between nurses and physiotherapists? What additional variables might this introduce (is it just a matter of different clinical discipline)? How would this additional comparison impact on the variables you have already identified?

Further reading

Sackett, D.L. and Wennberg, J.E. (1997) Choosing the best research design for each question. *British Medical Journal*, 315, 1636.

Websites

http://clem.mscd.edu/~davisj/prm2/correl1.html#1

http://psych.umb.edu/faculty/kogan/files/Handouts_CorrelationalDesigns.pdf

www.uiowa.edu/~resmeth/study_questions/sq-descrip-ccomp.html

19

Surveys

Key points

- Surveys are often wrongly assumed to be simple to carry out properly.
- Sampling technique and sample size are important in determining the margin of error in a survey.
- Survey designs are typically observational, but may also use experimental and quasi-experimental approaches.
- Decisions about question construction and questionnaire administration are fundamental to a successful survey.
- A review has revealed that some 'research folklore' guidelines about survey methods and question construction are not supported by empirical research.

Introduction

In our experience, the survey approach is the one most often attempted by students undertaking a research project as part of a course. Surveys are also a familiar part of our everyday lives, whether as part of advertising campaigns ('8 out of 10 owners said their cats preferred Cattoyum'), General Election TV coverage ('Over to Peter for news the

Research for Evidence-Based Practice in Healthcare, Second edition, by Robert Newell and Philip Burnard
© 2011 Robert Newell and Philip Burnard

results of our exit poll') or as a result of being stopped in the street and asked to participate in market research.

One unwanted effect of the familiarity of surveys is a common belief that surveys are easy to do. Unfortunately, this is not the case, and the successful completion of a survey actually requires a knowledge of aspects of almost each chapter in the quantitative section of this book (as well as, in some cases, aspects of the qualitative chapters, too!). In the next section, we will examine why this is so, before going on to describe issues which are particular to or especially important in the conducting of surveys.

Background issues in survey research

Different types of survey

In her excellent handbook on the topic, Fink (2003a,b,c) identifies four different types of survey: self-administration questionnaires, interviews, structured record reviews and structured observations. However, the last two of these approaches are usually not taken to be surveys by most researchers, because they may involve a number of different approaches. Indeed, record reviews and observations were excluded from a major review of research into survey approaches (McColl *et al.*, 2001). This is surprising, given that McColl *et al.*'s definition of a survey is: 'a set of scientific procedures for collecting information and making quantitative inferences about populations', a definition which certainly seems to include more than questionnaires and interviews. However, we have followed McColl *et al.*'s exclusion of record reviews and observations on the pragmatic grounds that we believe the definition of surveys in terms of question- and answer-based approaches is the one most generally understood in everyday life. That said, many of the issues raised in our discussion of questionnaires are equally applicable to the kind of recording that takes place in the context of document review or observation.

Surveys in brief

A set of scientific procedures for collecting information and making quantitative inferences about populations:

Self-administration questionnaires
Interviews
Structured record reviews
Structured observations

Sampling

One important element of the definition given above is the idea that quantitative inferences may be drawn about populations from the results of a survey. It follows from this that the surveyor must take account of the issues discussed in Chapter 6. Thus, surveyors will be aware of the need either to secure a random sample of the population being studied, or to be very circumspect in the kind of conclusions they seek to draw from their results. Essentially, the better the sample conforms to the population from which it is drawn, the more we can be confident that the findings within that sample are generalisable to the population.

Sample size is also important in this context. In Chapter 14, we saw how power in an experimental study was determined, in part, by the number of participants in the study. The same is true in surveys, although in a slightly different way. In surveys, we attempt to draw inferences from the study sample to its parent population, on the basis of the way in which participants respond to the survey questions. However, by their very nature, most survey samples will consist of only a small percentage of the study population. As a result of this, we may either find responses which appear significant or appear non-significant as a result of the fact that we have only surveyed these small numbers, in exactly the same way that a small number of coin tosses will usually give unequal numbers of heads and tails even if the coin is unbiased. Surveyors recognise this and often report the margin of error associated with the sample size they have used. This margin for error is, in essence, worked out by means of power calculations.

Reliability and validity

We discussed reliability and validity in detail in Chapters 6 and 13. In the context of surveys, the issue of external validity is mainly concerned with sampling, in the way we described in the previous section. Internal validity in surveys is principally concerned with how well the questions asked adequately investigate the concepts they claim to investigate, and, as a result, with how far the participant's answers accurately reflect what they think about the topic about which their views are being sought. Accordingly, other aspects of the survey situation (interviewer behaviour, time constraints, participant perception of the value or purpose of the study) are likewise issues which impact on internal validity.

Reliability in surveys is once again primarily concerned with instrument characteristics and researcher's behaviour. The first of these issues will be examined in detail later in this chapter. The second, researcher's behaviour, refers to how far the interviewer behaves in a consistent way in asking questions, clarifying misunderstandings, prompting respondents and recording responses. For example, if an interviewer always offered more clarification to female respondents than to males, it is easy to see how this would affect the reliability of the responses and lead to systematic bias in the responses of males versus females. There is also an issue of internal validity here, in that our confidence in the ability of the instrument *as delivered by such a researcher* to appropriately reflect the views of the respondents might be considerably compromised.

Survey designs

At first glance, it appears that all surveys are observational. However, if, for example, we gave respondents a questionnaire (say, a pre-test of knowledge of drug action), offered an intervention (teaching about drug actions), repeated the questionnaire, we are essentially undertaking a quasi-experiment using survey as the data collection method. Similarly, experimental use of a survey would also be possible.

Moreover, many survey instruments allow us to make subgroup comparisons, on the basis of identifying these subgroups from responses to particular items on the questionnaire (gender, qualification), then treating these subgroups as though they were different conditions of an independent variable, and seeing whether the responses of these subgroups to other questions on the questionnaire differ.

Surveys can be *cross-sectional*, where a sample is surveyed on a single occasion, or *longitudinal* where the same group is examined on two or more consecutive occasions. The example we gave of an experiment using survey methods is a longitudinal approach, but longitudinal surveys more usually simply examine uncontrolled, naturally occurring changes over time. Cross-sectional surveys very often involve examination of naturally occurring differences between subgroups at a single point in time.

Instrument design and question construction

Moser and Kalton (1993) presented a series of suggestions regarding the layout of questionnaires, which people conducting surveys have followed diligently ever since. These suggestions included the avoidance of vague, non-specific questions, hypothetical questions, leading questions, questions including technical and jargon words. The rationale behind these suggestions was essentially commonsensical, based on the notion that respondents will try and answer questions even if they do not understand them, will give misleading answers if they find questions difficult and will be subject to error based on lapses of memory and lack of awareness of their own attitudes. However, the research based on these assumptions and suggestions had only been established in the most rudimentary way, until a thorough review

---

Order:

Work from easier to harder questions
Use a logical order
Leave sensitive demographic details till the end

Question construction:

Make questions specific
Include a broad range of response alternatives
Alternatives should start with the least socially desirable response
For sensitive questions, use open-ended questions where possible; use wording
    which gives permission for a whole range of responses; embed threatening
    material within other material
Use open-ended questions sparingly
Avoid double-barrelled questions
State alternatives explicitly
Offer a middle response
Limit rating categories to no more than five points – use numerical scales for
    anything more

Figure 19.1   Guidelines for questionnaire construction.

undertaken by McColl *et al.* (2001). Most of our comments in the rest of this chapter draw heavily on that review and the original papers which are reviewed in it. Further suggestions for questionnaire wording are given in Figure 19.1.

The McColl *et al.* review examined studies testing most of the recommendations in Moser and Kalton and in Figure 19.1. Not surprisingly, given that most people would probably agree that these recommendations have a 'common sense' feel to them and intuitively seem very similar to how we would organise, for example, a conversation which sought to gain information from someone, most of them were supported.

However, the authors do note that a certain amount of caution should be applied, given that the majority of the studies into the relative merits of different ways of organising questionnaires were not conducted with health issues. Moreover, not all recommendations were supported. For example, it has been held that mixing negatively and positively worded questions reduces 'response set' (the tendency to tick consecutive questions with the same numbered response). Whist this might be so, there is an unwanted effect in reducing response validity, as accuracy of response is less for negatively worded items or mixed lists of positive and negative items. There is, therefore, potentially no advantage in mixing the polarity of items.

Likewise, the idea of grouping similar questions together makes intuitive sense, but is of doubtful value, because doing so creates context effects where responses to subsequent questions may be affected by responses to the preceding ones.

Finally, there is probably insufficient evidence upon which to base recommendations about the appearance of questionnaire materials, such as length, double- or single-sided printing, font size, nature and placement of instructions. In this context, it should be noted that this is because the amount of study given to these issues has been small, and absence of evidence of effect should not be taken as evidence of no effect. It is probably as well to offer participants well-presented questionnaires, even in the absence of consensus as to the importance of presentation.

Administration

Deciding how to administer your survey is a fundamental decision in survey research. There are essentially two alternatives: will the respondent be assisted in completing the instrument, or will they do so unaided. If you opt for assisted completion, you then have a choice between face-to-face interviews and telephone interviews. Most recently, there is also the option of internet-based assisted completion, which may be mediated by email access to an interviewer or via web-based context-specific material which offers more limited assistance (rather like an intelligent version of completion guidance notes). As with questionnaire construction, there have been advantages traditionally associated with one form of administration rather than another.

Response rates and representativeness. Assisted administration is usually associated with higher response rates, with less refusals, better access to a specific named individual and follow-up of that person. Finally, it is potentially more inclusive of people from different cultures or who have specific issues such as the inability to read.

Control of administration procedure. Assisted administration is usually claimed to give better control. For example, it deals best with long, complicated materials and allows the interviewer to explain difficulties with comprehension. It is also associated with lower non-response to individual items within a questionnaire.

By contrast, unaided response, typically via postal questionnaire is poor at all the above. However, it does have distinct advantages.

Interviewer bias. Postal questionnaires are regarded as being less open to the influence of the researcher. For example, there is no opportunity for the researcher to introduce bias either by way of the manner in which questions are asked or through providing more explanation (or different explanations) to some respondents than to others. One other important characteristic of the unaided interview is that the respondent is less likely to be influenced by social desirability considerations such as the desire to have the interviewer think well of them.

Practical constraints. Postal surveys have a huge advantage here for several reasons. There is no need to give staff special training (including possibly extensive training to reduce bias). The amount of staff time is small compared with either face-to-face or telephone interviews, and this again leads to cost reduction. If a suitable follow-up strategy can be designed, the amount of time taken to complete the survey can be comparatively modest, and large numbers of people can be reached during this small time period. This can lead to greater representativeness if issues of sampling bias can be overcome. Moreover, large samples usually suitable for more advanced statistical treatments.

However, despite the seemingly obvious nature of these supposed advantages and disadvantages, not all are supported by research evidence. The McColl *et al.* review found that evidence for some of the distinctions between assisted and unaided survey completion was equivocal. Their overall recommendation was that decisions regarding administration should be made on a survey-by-survey basis, taking account of study population, topic, sampling approach, volume and complexity of data to be collected, and resources available. No single approach to survey administration consistently outperforms another.

Thus, when face-to-face surveys, telephone surveys and postal questionnaires are compared, there is usually a higher response rate to face-to-face and telephone, but no consensus on whether face-to-face has higher response rate than telephone. Likewise, there is no unequivocal evidence that postal interviews are better than face-to-face at dealing with sensitive issues or social acceptability responses.

Enhancing response rate

We have already noted that face-to-face and telephone interviews are generally associated with higher response rates than postal surveys. However, there are a number of other things you can do to increase response rate which have been supported by research evidence, and some of these are very simple to achieve. They are summarised in Figure 19.2

Multiple contacts (follow-ups)
Pre-notification of the survey
Reply paid return envelope
Covering letter (traditional letters are better than novel approaches)
Cues to respondent indicating that completion time will be short
Topic which is timely, relevant and interesting
Incentives (especially financial!)

Figure 19.2 Increasing survey response rate.

Surprisingly, this list, which is once again taken from the comprehensive McColl *et al.* review, does not contain much of the research folklore advice to people wishing to conduct surveys. In particular, the following issues did not find support in empirical studies into enhancement of response rate: offering feedback about results; personalising letters to respondents; offers of confidentiality (surprisingly, these may actually *decrease response rate*); specification of a deadline; characteristics of the person conducting the survey.

Conclusion

As we noted at the beginning of this chapter, surveys are frequently conducted, especially in student projects, and are often thought of as an easy option. This is an unfortunate reputation, because the result is that they are often done badly, with inadequate preparation and poor execution. Given these circumstances, it is hardly surprising, also, that survey response rates are so low. A well-conducted survey is usually looking for a response rate around the 70% level, and researchers go to great care to maximise the likelihood of achieving this, especially in postal surveys, where the task is greater. Students and researchers working on individual projects can rarely expect this without considerable personal effort. However, where such an effort is made, the rewards are great in terms of the ability to reach large numbers of people and allow their opinions and experiences to be heard.

Review Questions

What are the four main types of survey data collection?
What issues surrounding questionnaire construction have been supported by research?
What are the main issues of concern in survey administration?

Exercise

We regularly receive surveys through the mail, either as part of courses we are attending, through work, or from commercial companies. Next time you receive one, read it in conjunction with this chapter and assess how far the person conducting the survey has met the criteria we have described here. In particular, look at the way the questions are worded and assess each one for clarity.

References

Fink, A. (2003a) *The Survey Handbook*. London: Sage.

Fink, A. (2003b) *How to Ask Survey Questions*. London: Sage.

Fink, A. (2003c) *How to Manage, Analyse and Interpret Survey Data*. London: Sage.

McColl, E., Jacoby, A., Thomas, L., Soutter, J., Bamford, C., Steen, N., Thomas, R., Harvey, E., Garratt, A. and Bond, J. (2001) Design and use of question-naires: a review of best practice applicable to surveys of health service staff and patients. *Health Technology Assessment*, 5(31).

Moser, C. and Kalton, G. (1993) *Survey Methods in Social Investigation*. Aldershot: Dartmouth.

Further reading

Oppenheim, A.N. (1992) *Questionnaire Design, Interviewing and Attitude Measurement*, 2nd edn. London: Pinter.

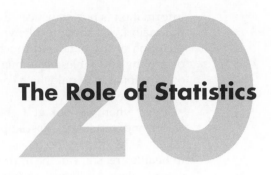

The Role of Statistics

Why do I need to know about statistical tests?

If you take a look at any paper published in medical and healthcare journals, you will probably find that something like 95% or more of the

Research for Evidence-Based Practice in Healthcare, Second edition, by Robert Newell and Philip Burnard
© 2011 Robert Newell and Philip Burnard

information is non statistical. Even when you reach the results section, the majority of these results will amount to little more than basic description of the data, and much of this will be displayed in the form of graphs and tables. This might lead us to suspect that the amount of additional material which complicated statistics convey is of limited importance. Not so.

Even when we look at a graph or table, it is known that observer errors and systematic biases operate (see Chapter 16). The more complicated the display becomes, the greater the likelihood of error, and in healthcare, some of the information we seek to communicate is very complicated. An understanding of statistics can help us to avoid these errors and biases.

More than that, there is some information which cannot be conveyed by visual inspection alone. Probably the example you will be most familiar with is results of studies of treatment effectiveness. Imagine two treatments for fatigue have been compared. Fifty patients have been offered an exercise programme, whilst another 50 have been given cognitive behaviour therapy (CBT) – a popular treatment for chronic fatigue. The results graph shows 30 of the exercise group have improved, compared with 35 in the CBT group. Most of us would recognise that a difference of five between the two groups does not necessarily represent a difference between the two treatments. If we also know that patients in the CBT group we slightly more severely affected at the start of treatment, the picture becomes more complicated. Trying to convey all this information in a meaningful, interpretable way by showing raw data is nigh on impossible.

What are statistics for

Statistics have a bad reputation because they are seen as difficult, and not without reason. They are associated with maths, a subject which is renowned as a problem for people at school, and many people carry maths fears with them throughout their adult lives. Yet, the amount of mathematical knowledge you require to be a statistics *user* (not a statistician!) is actually very small. In the rest of this chapter, we will see that most understanding of statistics in healthcare, at the level a clinician needs, requires not mathematical knowledge and expertise, but knowing a few important basic concepts and getting to grips with some of the special language used in the field.

The first thing to be aware of in approaching this topic is that statistics really are useful. For our purposes, their uses can be divided into two categories: descriptive and inferential. Happily, these two categories exactly state what they set out to do, for descriptive statistics are designed to describe data, usually, by summarising important characteristics of it, whilst inferential statistics allow us to make predictions from the data – in other words to draw inferences from it.

Both of these activities, describing/summarising and predicting/inferring represent attempts on the part of statistical approaches to make sense of the mass of raw data with which we are often confronted at the end of a research study. In other words, the central aim of all statistical work is to *simplify*. If this seems unlikely, consider the above example of the two treatments for fatigue. At the end of the study, we would have at least 200 data points (50 pre- and post-treatment scores for the each treatment group). Simple descriptive statistics allow us to present *all the important aspects* of those data points in two figures: the mean difference between the two groups and the difference between the spread of the two groups. We will talk about these two terms later. For now, the basic principle is that statistics can be an ally in understanding large quantities of data. That is what statistics are for.

Basic ideas: visual displays, levels of data and statistics

Perhaps the most common way to present and simplify data is through the use of graphs and tables, although, as we noted above, these are not without their shortcomings, and may be difficult to interpret, particularly where large amounts of data are presented. It is very common for students to be advised to include graphs and tables in their reports, because these forms of visual display break up the text and add interest and impact. However, these are not adequate reasons for the use of displays. We recommend that graphs and tables be used only when they add to clarity and simplicity of the data to be presented.

The main types of graphs you are likely to meet are histograms and bar charts. Both plot frequency of response, but histograms are used for continuous data, whilst bar charts are used for categorical data.

This brings us to a first important general notion in understanding statistics: the idea of levels of measurement. There are four such levels, each of which relates to a different way in which numbers are being used. For statistical purposes, the most important distinction is probably between continuous data, which consists of three levels (ratio, interval and ordinal), and categorical data, which consists of one level (nominal or categorical).

Dealing with nominal level data first, this level of data is the most limited in terms of the range of statistical tests which can be applied to it, mainly because, with nominal level data, the numbers used are really codes for different categories of things. Although this sounds confusing, we do this kind of thing all the time. In the example of two treatments for fatigue, for example, we might refer to exercise as treatment 1 and CBT as treatment 2. Although the treatments are *called* 1 and 2, this does not mean that 1 is smaller than 2 in the same way that, for example, 1 cm is smaller than 2 cm. The numbers, in this context, are simply names to denote particular things. As another example, we might be interested in whether people preferred chocolate or fruit as a dessert, and enter these into a database with codes 1 for chocolate and 2 for fruit. Once again, all that is being done here is the arbitrary assignment of a number to each of the desserts as a shorthand *name* for it. The word *nominal* itself derives from the latin word *nomen*, meaning a name.

For statistical purposes, only a few tests are suitable for nominal level data, because, basically, the only sort of statistical examination we can do with such data is to observe and compare the frequencies with which data occur (e.g. how many people prefer chocolate and how many prefer fruit). Relatively few statistical tests deal with frequency of response alone. Most deal with the size of response also (e.g. how much each person prefers chocolate or fruit). These tests require the use of one form or another of continuous data.

Ordinal level data refers to data which can be meaningfully placed in rank order. If we ask people how much they like their dessert (5 = very much, 4 = somewhat, 3 = indifferent, 2 = not much, 1 = not at all) we are now using numbers to indicate differences in the amount of response. In this example, we are saying people who score 5 like their dessert more than those who score 4, people who score 4 like it more than those who score 3 and so on. However, it is not the case that those who score 4 like their dessert twice as much as those who score 2. Nor is it the case that the difference between scores of 5 and 4 is the same as the difference between scores of 4 and 3. If we translate the numbers back to the words they represent, this becomes obvious. Is the difference between liking something 'very much' and 'somewhat' the same as the difference between liking it 'somewhat' and being 'indifferent' to it. Who can say? Therefore, although the data are ranked, there is no sense in which the intervals between the ranks are necessarily the same. In consequence, statistical tests used with ordinal level data work only with the ranks of the data, without making assumptions about equality of intervals.

Interval level data allows us to make exactly this assumption. Typically, characteristics of the physical world conform to interval level data. Thus, body temperature, foot size, blood values and so on are all at interval level. One degree centigrade really is half of two degrees on that scale, which is really half of four degrees and so on. Interval level data is extremely flexible in that it allows the use of sophisticated statistical tests which treat the numbers *as numbers* rather than as categories or ranks.

Finally, ratio level data is essentially a variant of interval level data, with the exception that ratio level data possesses an absolute zero. In consequence, ratios of differences between different scores on such variables are independent of the scale used. Weight and height are examples of this. For most practical purposes, the theoretical differences between interval and ratio level data do not affect the statistical tests to be used in the healthcare context.

> **Increasing levels of data offer increasingly complex and sensitive possibilities for analysis**
>
> Nominal level data – names (categories) of things
> Ordinal level data – ranks (ranked categories of things)
> Interval level data – data where the ranks are at equal intervals (numbers)
> Ratio level data – data where there is an absolute zero number possible

Descriptive statistics

As we said earlier, descriptive statistics do no more than describe the data in a way which is accessible to the reader. Most often this will begin with a record of the frequency with which particular responses occurred and the magnitude of those responses. This is not, however, essential, and some research reports, particularly those with large amounts of complex descriptive data will omit frequency counts and go straight for measures of *central tendency and spread.*

As you might expect from the previous section, different levels of data are associated with different measures of central tendency and spread. Because nominal level data is concerned solely with frequencies, the *mode* is the appropriate measure of central tendency, because it is the most frequently occurring value.

For ordinal level data, we use the *median* as the estimate of central tendency. The median is the middle ranking number in the data set. To measure spread around this central measure, we use quartiles and centiles. These tell us, respectively, the value below which each 25% or each 10% of the data fall.

With interval level data, the mean is the measure of central tendency, and is familiar to almost everyone from school, where it was often referred to the average. It is calculated by adding all the values together and dividing the result by the number of values. For measures of spread, we have a choice of at least three different measures. Most simply, the range is the distance between the highest and lowest values. This conveys considerable extra information about the dataset. The second such measure of spread, the *variance* gives more, however. Whilst the method if its calculation is beyond the scope of this chapter, the resulting figure tells us how much, on average, the values in the dataset vary from the mean. Thus, if we know that a dataset has a mean of 6 and a variance of 2, we know that the *average* amount for the values in the dataset differ from 6 is 2, in other words, between 4 and 8. Please note that this is *not* the same as saying the range is from 4 to 8, because an average difference of between 4 and 8 could arise from a considerable number of raw scores, including ones above and below these numbers. Knowing this helps us from being distracted by outlying values. Finally, the *standard deviation* is the square root of the variance. This may seem a bit obscure, but the standard deviation is probably the most widely reported measure of spread. This is because it is related to the *normal distribution*, a construct which helps us to describe large datasets in detail and underpins much statistically testing involving interval level data.

> **Central tendency, spread and the distribution curve**
>
> Between them, a measure of central tendency (mean, median, mode) and a measure of spread (variance, standard deviation, range) give a concise summary picture of the whole dataset.
> The distribution curve shows the shape of this distribution.

Normal distribution

The normal distribution curve is a bell-shaped curve of frequencies of responses (see Figure 20.1) to which many physical, psychological and social phenomena correspond. The curve in Figure 20.1 shows that only a few values are either extremely small or extremely large. The vast majority of values are clustered around the measure of central tendency. At the midpoint on the normal distribution curve are the mean, median and mode. The two vertical lines drawn on each side of the mean line represent standard deviations. Taking the curve as a whole, 95% of the values in any normally distributed dataset lie within

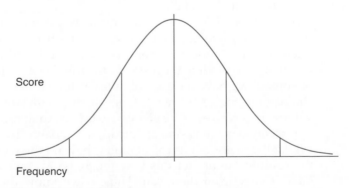

Figure 20.1   The normal distribution curve.

two standard deviations above and below the mean. So, if we say a dataset has a mean value of 10 with a standard deviation of 3, we are saying that 95% of the values lie between 1 and 16. This is a powerful, simple and accurate description of the data.

Parametric and non-parametric statistical tests

Parametric tests make a number of assumptions about the data for which they are used (the parameters to which the data should conform). The first of these is that the level of the data is interval or ratio. This is because parametric tests treat the numbers as if the intervals between them were equal, rather than simply ranks or categories. The second parameter to which the data should conform is that it should be normally distributed. This is because comparisons between the two groups are based on the premise that there should be a certain amount of separation between the distribution curves of the two groups for us to have confidence that they really represent two different populations, rather than subsets of a single one. This assertion is harder to justify using parametric tests if the data are not normally distributed (see Figure 20.2). Finally, the data must possess homogeneity of variance – in other words, the variance within the groups being analysed must be roughly similar. If we know the data are normally distributed *and* the variances are similar, then the only characteristic of the samples which can give rise to a difference is the means of those samples – the thing we are generally comparing in parametric tests.

Having said all this, it should be noted that some researchers and statisticians deny the distinction we have just made between parametric and non-parametric tests. They argue that the important difference is between continuous data and categorical data, and that this distinction should guide our choice of statistical tests. Non-statisticians,

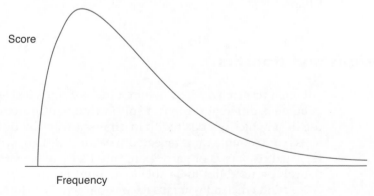

Figure 20.2 A non-normal distribution.

however, are probably best sticking with the conservative rationale for test selection we have given here.

Inferential statistics

Statistical significance

In speaking of statistical significance, we are asserting that a particular event or response would be unlikely to have occurred by chance. If it did not occur by chance, we assume that it was caused by some effect of the independent variable on the dependent variable, or some interaction between two or more variables. The criterion set in science for statistical significance is <5% (probability of $p < 0.05$). Both these statements say that the event or response would not have occurred by chance as frequently as one time in 20. This is a purely arbitrary convention, and circumstances might occur in which we would wish to set this criterion higher. Given the durability of the convention, however, our reasons for changing the criterion would have to be very strong indeed.

This means that every time we get a statistically significant result at the 5% level, we would have arrived at such a result one time in 20 by chance (called a *type I error*). Conversely, every time we get a non-significant result at the 5% level we have missed, by chance, a result that actually did not occur by chance (called a *type II error*). Moreover, if we run several tests on a dataset, we increase the chance that we will make a type I error. If we run two tests, it is two in 20, if few run three tests, it is three in 20 and so on. The best rule for avoiding type I error is to have a strong rationale for each test you run, and do not run any others. In other words, no fishing trips in the data. The best rule for avoiding a type II error is to increase sample size, because risk of type II error is related to sample size. Small studies are *underpowered* (see Chapter 14).

Designs and statistics

Different research designs require different statistical approaches. This is because different designs result in different sources of variation in the data, which are dealt with in different ways by different statistical tests. For example, in a repeated measures design, we know that the repeated responses of participants are likely to be correlated. The statistical test used has to be able to account for this naturally occurring correlation when allowing us to consider whether differences observed are statistically significant.

Testing for differences
Repeated measures designs (before–after studies):
   Interval level data (comparison of means): two groups – related t-test; three or more groups – one-way ANOVA
   Ordinal level data (comparison of ranks): two groups – Wilcoxon test; three or more groups – Friedman test.
   Nominal level data (comparison of frequencies) – McNemar's test
Independent groups designs:
   Repeated measures designs (before–after studies):
   Interval level data (comparison of means): two groups – unrelated t-test; three or more groups – one-way ANOVA
   Ordinal level data (comparison of ranks): two groups – Mann–Whitney *U* test; three or more groups – Kruskall–Wallis test
   Nominal level data (comparison of frequencies) – Chi-square test

Controlling for unwanted differences
Univariate and multivariate analysis of variance and covariance (ANOVA and MANOVA)

Analysing interactions
Univariate and multivariate analysis of variance and covariance (ANCOVA and MANCOVA)
Regression analysis

Tests for correlation
Interval level data: Pearson's product moment co-efficient
Ordinal level data: Spearman's rho
Nominal level data: contingency co-efficient

Figure 20.1   Common research designs and their most used statistical tests.

Broadly speaking, this same issue accounts for the fact that different statistical tests are used in tests for difference from those used in correlational testing, and in tests for differences or interactions between two groups from those used in the examination if differences or interactions between three or more groups.

The same proposition applies if we want to examine the causal effect of two different variables on a person's response (factorial designs – see Chapter 15). The statistical test must be able to tell us the effect of each individual independent variable, *plus* the interaction of those variables. Because of the complexity of the design, data and statistical analysis involved factorial studies and their analyses usually involve the use of interval level data.

A guide to the main tests used in testing for differences and interactions is shown in Figure 20.1.

Estimation and confidence intervals

All the above discussion has taken place in the context of hypothesis testing in research (see Chapter 14). As you will recall, this is an all or nothing approach in which an assertion (hypothesis) is either rejected or accepted, and the statistical tests described here are the means whereby we can have confidence in making this judgement. However, we also touched, in Chapter 14, on an alternative way of examining relationships between sample and population. In estimation, we are concerned with qualitative judgements about the level of relationship between our sample and population. The main way of assessing this is by the use of confidence intervals, which tell us the range of values which we believe represent the upper and lower borders of the population being considered, typically, with 95% confidence that these are accurate estimates. If the value for our sample lies within these limits, we can be confident that the sample is truly part of the population. By extension, if we know the confidence intervals of the *difference* between two groups, and our result is between these we can be confident that this is an accurate estimation of the difference between the groups. Moreover, the smaller the space between the two confidence intervals, the greater the likelihood that our value is an accurate estimate of the population. Knowing that our value of 10 lies between confidence intervals of 8 and 12 gives us a lot more knowledge about the representativeness of the result than knowing that it lies between values of 1 and 50. For more discussion of confidence intervals, see Altman *et al.* (2001).

Is this really all I need to know?

In your clinical practice, this degree of statistical knowledge will see you a long way. In fact, it is probably more than you need to know. However, if you have managed to get to the end of this chapter, you probably have at least some interest in knowing more (or you already know something about statistics!), and will have realised we have only scratched the surface of this fascinating subject.

For example, in Figure 20.1 we have not described the use of ANOVA, MANOVA, ANCOVA or MANCOVA because their use requires not only some statistical knowledge, but also a relatively sophisticated grasp of research design and its conceptual underpinnings. Similarly, we have not ventured to describe the use of factor analysis in the construction of psychological measures or the way in which multiple regression can explore correlations between many variables in large datasets and use some of these variables to predict how others will behave. All these approaches have much to offer the clinical practitioner and are, to a greater or lesser extent, based on the concepts we have introduced in this chapter. The recommended reading will guide you some of the ways in increasing your understanding of both the basics, and these more complex applications. In this chapter, we have deliberately stayed away from giving any figure work at all. We believe if you want to get to grips with quantitative data analysis, you have to do some figure work – not to be a statistician, but to be a knowledgeable *statistics user.* Computer packages will do all the figure work for you, but doing some of the basics by hand (at least once!) is the only real way of getting an understanding of some of the concepts statisticians use.

Review questions

What are the main purposes of descriptive and inferential statistics?
What do we mean by statistical significance?
Why are there different statistical tests associated with different levels of data and different research designs?

Exercise

Get hold of three pieces of quantitative research relevant to your current clinical work. Examine the statistics section whilst re-reading this chapter, and try to get to grips with what the numbers are telling you. Denis Anthony's book (below) will offer you more guidance if you need it.

Reference

Altman, D.G., Machin, D., Bryant, T.N. and Gardner, M.J. (2001) *Statistics with Confidence.* London: BMJ Books.

Further reading

Altman, D.G. (1990) *Practical Statistics for Medical Research.* London: Chapman & Hall.

Anthony, D. (1999) *Understanding Advanced Statistics: A Guide for Nurses and Health Care Researchers.* Edinburgh: Churchill Livingstone.

Bland, M. (2002) *An Introduction to Medical Statistics.* Oxford: Oxford University Press.

Clegg, F. (1983) *Simple Statistics.* Cambridge: Cambridge University Press.

Website

http://hsc.uwe.ac.uk/dataanalysis/quantWhat.asp

SECTION 4
Appraisal, Dissemination and Implementation

Evidence-Based Practice and Clinical Effectiveness

Key points

- Research aims to add to the evidence to inform clinical practice.
- Evidence-based practice (EBP) and clinical effectiveness are related terms, but clinical effectiveness has the narrower focus.
- EBP is a process involving: asking answerable questions, finding evidence, appraising the evidence, applying evidence to practice, evaluating performance of EBP.
- The hierarchy of evidence runs from most to least trustworthy on the basis of freedom from bias.
- EBP is intended to enhance clinical decision making, not replace it.

Evidence and clinical practice

One of the major purposes of research is to add to the body of evidence in a particular field of knowledge. In practical disciplines such as medicine and healthcare, it is usually expected that this knowledge

Research for Evidence-Based Practice in Healthcare, Second edition, by Robert Newell and Philip Burnard
© 2011 Robert Newell and Philip Burnard

will support practice. We want the best possible outcomes for patients, and so engage in research in order to discover how to achieve these outcomes. This does not mean only research into which treatments work best, but also studies of, for example, patient characteristics, processes of disease, illness and recovery, the organisation and care. Because all these issues potentially affect patient outcomes, all are legitimate sources of study in a clinical discipline and, as a result, potential sources of evidence according to which that discipline should be carried out.

Surprisingly, very little of our care is evidence based. This is a particular problem for us in the healthcare professions other than medicine for two reasons. First, as the largest clinical group providing healthcare to patients, we have the most contact with them. As a result, our opportunities to influence the course of their illness and recovery are enormous. If our care is not evidence based, the potential for us to harm them rises accordingly. Second, we lack the traditional power base of medicine (whose care, incidentally, also often lacks an evidence base). Because of this, it is easy for other disciplines to impose upon us their own ideas of how care should be organised. Evidence for our clinical practice represents one way in which we can assert ourselves on behalf of our patients.

This is not to say that no evidence is available. Indeed, we have only to look at the internet to see how the availability and extent of information (including information on health matters) has exploded in recent years. Unfortunately, there is no necessary relationship between quantity and quality; nor is there a relationship between either of these things and use. In medicine, the majority of general practitioners read for about an hour a week, and the majority of their reading is from textbooks. This is in spite of the information explosion. None of this is surprising, given that clinicians are very busy with the practical work of consultation and treatment. The move towards evidence-based care is an attempt to put information at the heart of healthcare and make it usable to clinicians.

What are EBP and clinical effectiveness?

These two terms are often used virtually interchangeably to refer to any process of using evidence to enhance patient care. However, we take the view that clinical effectiveness has a slightly narrower focus, being essentially about patient health gain through the implementation of interventions supported by a body of evidence for effectiveness. Indeed, the original National Health Service Executive description seems to support this definition.

NHS definition of clinical effectiveness

'The extent to which specific clinical interventions when deployed in the field for a particular patient or population do what they are intended to do, that is, maintain and improve health and secure the greatest possible health gain from the available resources' (NHSE, 1996).

EBP is also a process (part of whose aims may be the deployment of the most clinically effective interventions), best viewed as a lifelong educational exercise which carries on the whole time one is in clinical practice. The process consists of the following five stages, which can be aimed at meeting the health needs of an individual or group:

Stages in EBP

(1) asking answerable questions
(2) finding the best available evidence
(3) appraising the evidence for its validity and applicability
(4) applying the results of this appraisal in clinical practice
(5) evaluating performance of EBP

In EBP, then, evidence of clinical effectiveness is one element of the process. This is combined with the clinician's own expertise to produce a solution to a clinical question in a way which is relevant to the patient's individual needs and preferences. It is this point which has often been misunderstood and led critics of EBP and clinical effectiveness to argue that these are mechanistic approaches to care which remove clinician and patient choice. Unfortunately, the way in which the EBP movement has been interpreted by some Governmental institutions has often led to just such inflexibility, but this is precisely the opposite of what is intended by proponents of the use of the evidence-based approach. Evidence is intended to inform and support clinical judgement, not to supplant it, and comes from many sources other than published research studies (e.g. laboratory tests, the patient's own accounts). The clinician's job is to process these difference sources in a holistic way in order to create unique solutions in patient care. Nevertheless, research evidence is an important element in the whole picture, and one which has often been overlooked in the past.

The process of EBP in practice

In this section, we will unpick the five stages in the EBP process to show how it can be applied to patient problems.

During earlier chapters we have already discovered that asking a well-defined research question is not necessarily easy. The same thing applies to clinical questions. Each patient presents us with a set of unique challenges. For example, the district nurse working with a patient with leg ulcers who is also suffering from fatigue and depression, and is unable to get to the shops or her social club, is dealing with an individual with multifaceted issues in the physical, psychological and social spheres. The first step in addressing these with the support of evidence-based literature is to ask a question (or series of questions) which identify both the problem areas and how the literature might assist us. These questions need to be sufficiently specific to guide us through the various aspects of the person's difficulties. We will take fatigue as the issue to be addressed here.

Question formulation

One well-established route through question formulation is described on the Canadian Centre for Evidence Base Medicine (CEBM) website, from which much of the following EBP process description has been derived. The clinician specifies the question by considering: the *patient or problem; the possible intervention; the comparison intervention; the desired outcome.*

> In the case of fatigue, the answerable question might look as follows: For a 70 year old woman with fatigue (patient & problem), can cognitive-behaviour therapy (CBT) (intervention) decrease fatigue or increase activity (outcomes) compared with no treatment (comparison intervention)?

Naturally, the sensitive clinician will have discussed the desired outcomes with the patient beforehand. However, the key point here is that appropriate question formulation guides the next step.

Finding the evidence

For the purpose of this discussion, we are only examining research literature, but the clinician will also take into account tests, the patient's own views, and the views of carers in determining how to proceed. We recommend using a hierarchy of evidence (see final section) to guide this stage in the EBP process. The hierarchy runs from most reliable to least reliable evidence. As a rule of thumb, if evidence exists at the highest level, it is not necessary to search below that level. In this case, the sources of evidence are electronic databases in the first instance (see Chapter 4).

In fact, a systematic review of treatment for chronic fatigue exists, and is highly relevant, even though it is not specific to intervention with fatigue in leg ulcer patients (Interventions for the Management of CFS/ME [NHS Centre for Reviews and Dissemination, 2006]) which suggests that CBT is effective in chronic fatigue. A clinician working with evidence-based care might feel justified in extending these results to a leg ulcer patient with fatigue.

Appraising the evidence

The amount of work that has gone into constructing a systematic review means that we can have reasonable confidence in its findings. However, criteria exist which allow us to critically evaluate such reviews (available from the CEBM website and others) if we are doubtful about its findings and have time to do so. Where no systematic review exists, the burden of appraisal falls more squarely on the shoulders of the clinician.

Applying the evidence

Application of evidence relies on a combination of one's own clinical abilities, the availability of resource and acceptability to patients. For example, if the nurse in this example had attended a course in cognitive-behaviour therapy (CBT), they might feel confident to apply the CBT approach to fatigue with this patient. If not, they might be thinking of referring on to a cognitive-behaviour therapist who did possess such skills. All these courses of action should be negotiated with the patient in accordance with their own views. Finally, the clinician should attempt to evaluate the success of applying the evidence with this patient.

Evaluating one's own performance

Surprisingly, little of this is concerned with evaluating performance of the clinical intervention. Rather, it falls from the earlier stages of the EBP process. The clinician attempts to self-evaluate in terms of how well they have used the EBP approach with this patient, looking at all stages of the process. Training needs may emerge from this, some of which may be therapeutic whilst others related directly to the conduct of EBP. In this example, the nurse might recognise a need to gain better critical appraisal skills in the future, in case she encounters patient problems for which systematic reviews are not available or are highly equivocal.

The nature of evidence to support practice

In view of the great explosion of information availability, and range of quality of this information, it is useful to be able to grade this information. In the previous section, we mentioned the hierarchy of evidence. This notion of different levels of evidence, associated with different levels of trustworthiness for clinicians is one way of grading evidence which has found general acceptance in healthcare is the notion of levels of evidence (Figure 21.1).

We believe it is possible to add two further, even lower sources of evidence: opinions of our professional colleagues (who may or may not be experts in their fields) and evidence from our own professional experience. These two lowest levels are enticing because of their easy availability and their assumed trustworthiness (after all, if you cannot trust your own experience or your friends and colleagues, who can you trust?). We do not say you should *necessarily* distrust either, but offer the warning that simply because a source of information is easy to find does not necessarily make it reliable. Psychologists even tell us that our own memories for events are open to systematic bias! Individual opinions need to be taken account of, but within the broader range of sources of evidence. Apart from anything else, it is an act of professional arrogance (and probably unethical) to prefer one's personal opinion over evidence from a systematic review which may have taken a large team of academics and clinicians years to compile and maintain.

This is, at root, the reason why the levels of evidence presented in Figure 21.1 are organised hierarchically, with level 1 being the most reliable and level 5 the least. Systematic reviews of randomised controlled trials are the least susceptible to bias of all the levels of evidence

---

(1) Strong evidence from at least one systematic review
(2) Strong evidence from at least one randomised controlled trial of appropriate size
(3) Evidence from well-designed non-randomised trials
(4) Evidence from well-designed non-experimental studies from more than one research group or centre
(5) Expert authority opinion or reports of expert committees
    (Adapted from Muir Gray, 1997)

Figure 21.1   Levels of evidence.

because at each stage (study search, selection, appraisal, study methodology of each contributing study) the researchers have taken care to use methods into which as little bias as possible has crept to diminish our confidence in the validity of the findings. Randomised trials represent the next-least biased, and so on, for the same reason. This does not mean these higher levels in the hierarchy of evidence are perfect, just that they are more trustworthy than those lower down. As busy clinicians, this is important because it means that, if a systematic review exists on a particular clinical topic, we rarely have to read a dozen or so studies of that topic in order to inform our practice.

Criticisms of EBP

Earlier in this chapter, we noted that some clinicians have felt EBP had the potential to erode their clinical autonomy and judgement, but that this has never been the intention. Rather, EBP is intended to enhance that judgement. Clinicians have often voiced a related criticism – that EBP is not patient-centred, because it relies on the general applicability of treatments, rather than tailoring interventions to individual client problems. We hope that our outline and example of the application of EBP has to some extent disarmed that criticism. Our own belief is that the application of tried and tested treatments is one of the most patient-centred things a clinician can do. Certainly, applying treatments which do not have an adequate evidence base must be the least, because, without knowledge of evidence, the clinician cannot give an adequate rationale for treatment to the patient, and without that rationale, the patient cannot make an informed choice. We regard adequate evidence as a prerequisite for patient-centredness.

Other common criticisms of EBP include the notion that it is a cost-cutting or treatment rationing exercise. EBP is certainly concerned with cost effectiveness, but this is not the same as cost-cutting. The rationale behind cost-effective treatment is that the pool of money will always be finite, and for every treatment you perform you lose the opportunity to perform another. Thus, it is important to choose the one with the best evidence behind it, including evidence of cost effectiveness. As with any effective approach, EBP, can be misused, and institutions may choose to do so. However, with EBP the decisions taken are more transparent and, therefore, more open to question by vigilant clinicians and patients.

Finally, it has been suggested that EBP is restricted to the use of randomised controlled trials. However, this is not so. EBP often makes extensive use of these studies for the reasons we touched on above, primarily because these studies are best at demonstrating the effectiveness of clinical interventions. Nevertheless, the entire range of research studies is considered in EBP, including non-experimental studies and qualitative research. The only criterion is that the evidence generated by a study is sufficiently methodologically robust to allow the study's use in guiding care.

Indeed, this is perhaps the best way to think of EBP, as an educational process to assist and guide the HCP care rather than determine it.

Review questions

What are the five stages in EBP?
What are the five levels of evidence?
What are the main criticisms of EBP? How convincing do you find them?

Exercise

Using the five stages in the EBP process, take a recent example of your own care and apply the process to finding best evidence. Consider how you would apply this evidence in the future.

References

Muir Gray, J.A. (1997) *Evidence Based Healthcare: How to Make Health Policy and Management Decisions*. Edinburgh: Churchill Livingstone.

NHS Centre for Dissemination and Reviews (2006) Effective treatments for CFS/ME. CRD Report 35. York: University of York.

Further reading

DiCenso, A., Ciliska, D., Cullum, N. and Guyatt, G. (2003) *Evidence Based Nursing: A Guide to Clinical Practice*. London: Mosby.

NHS Executive (1996) *Promoting Clinical Effectiveness: A Framework for Action in and through the NHS*. London: Department of Health.

Sackett, D.L., Straus, S., Richardson, W.S., Rosenberg, W. and Haynes, R.B. (2005) *Evidence Based Medicine: How to Practice and Teach EBM*. Edinburgh: Churchill Livingstone.

Websites

http://www.york.ac.uk/inst/crd/CRD_Reports/crdreport35_summ.pdf

http://www.bmj.com/cgi/content/full/312/7023/71?view=long&pmid=8555924

http://www.ncbi.nlm.nih.gov/pubmed/8555924

http://www.cebm.utoronto.ca/practise/formulate/pg2.htm

http://www.medicine.ox.ac.uk/bandolier/

Critical Evaluation of Research Reports

22

Key points

- The ability to weigh evidence is a required skill for competent practitioners.
- A good literature review should critically examine the literature and set the current study in that context.
- The method section should be detailed and demonstrate appropriate choices.
- Different specific methodological issues are associated with qualitative and quantitative research.
- The results section should be clear.
- Quantitative results should distinguish between significant and non-significant results.
- Qualitative results should avoid claims as to generalisability.
- The discussion section should set the results in the context of the literature, implications for practice and further research.
- Study weaknesses should be honestly and comprehensively reported.

Research for Evidence-Based Practice in Healthcare, Second edition, by Robert Newell and Philip Burnard
© 2011 Robert Newell and Philip Burnard

Introduction

Critical appraisal of published work is enormously important in the NHS for several reasons. First, whilst very few people working in the NHS will themselves carry out research, almost all will directly or indirectly utilise research findings. Of these, very few will themselves examine and review more than a tiny number of primary sources of research findings (e.g. journal articles reporting the findings of research studies). Most clinicians are busy people, and rely heavily on synopses of the research studies which have generated the evidence for their practice.

Typically, these synopses are made available either in review articles, abstracting journals or textbooks. These sources of information, at their best, are underpinned by skilled appraisal of the primary research studies. In this chapter, we will examine how such appraisal is carried out. As a consequence, you will have an awareness of the process which has occurred in the generation of the key texts and guidelines which direct much of your work, but will also be equipped to begin to appraise primary research findings for yourself. Moreover, if you are undertaking almost any course in healthcare, evaluation of published research will almost certainly be the basis of one or more assignments, as well as forming part of almost every other assignment, because the ability to weigh evidence is regarded as a crucial skill for competent practitioners. Different institutions will have varying specific guidelines for these assignments, but the general guidelines we have presented here should prepare you to undertake sound evaluation of published research in pretty much any context.

Much of the material which follows here is in summary and note form. This is for the very good reason that appraisal of published research requires a thorough understanding of the process and practice of research, and this is precisely what we have tried to give you during the earlier chapters of this book. We can summarise this by saying that a competent research paper is one which follows all the guidelines laid out in these earlier chapters, and presents to you, the reader, a coherent account of how it has done so. Accordingly, we will summarise key issues from previous chapters as they apply to reading a research report, but also note additional criteria which should be met to make it clear to the reader that these key issues have been addressed by the researchers.

Most particularly, we will try to help you in forming and justifying judgments about those elements of research reports where guidelines are less formalised. For example, the criteria for judging appropriateness of method are, pretty much, a reflection of our discussions in previous chapters, but how do you judge the quality of a literature review or the usefulness of a discussion section?

One important point that we ask you to bear in mind from the outset is that what we are describing here is a set of guidelines as to the *best possible* conduct and reporting of research. Almost every report you read will fall short of these best practices in one way or another, and we freely admit that much of our own research has fallen short. This is because research (particularly health research) takes place in the real world, and a balance often has to be struck between methodological considerations and practical constraints. Practical constraints almost always win out in any struggle of this kind, because if we did not, as researchers, pay heed to such constraints, little research would ever be done. In consequence, almost all research has flaws. It is your job, as an appraiser of research, to come to a judgement as to how far these flaws affect our confidence in what the researcher asserts has been discovered in the study. In summary, do not dismiss research because it is flawed, but consider it in the light of those flaws and judge its merit accordingly.

Reading the paper

Title

A good title tells you exactly what a paper is about and nothing else. There is a trend, as we suggested in Chapter 2, particularly in popular and professional journals towards catchy, attention-grabbing titles. For the purpose of reviewing research these are of little value. The fact that a title is attention-grabbing tells you nothing about the quality of the work contained therein, and, quite possible, little about the content either. Is a paper entitled 'Falls in older people: the way forward' a discussion of Government policy on falls prevention, a description of a hospital's approach to rehabilitation, an account of a novel treatment approach, a plea for better resourcing or something else? The title, therefore, should tell you, as the reader, exactly what to expect.

More than this, a good title helps in the process of searching the literature, and for this reason it is good practice to refer to a thesaurus of the kind used by most databases, in order to increase the likelihood that people searching the literature will be likely to access a paper if it is relevant to their needs. The use of keywords likewise increases this likelihood.

Authors

Some guides to critical evaluation still suggest that reviewers comment on the authorship of a paper, looking at how experienced the authors are in the field and the extent to which they are regarded as expert. We see no reason at all to follow this advice, which perhaps springs from a misplaced regard for the value of authority rather than argument in scholarship. After all, many important discoveries have been made by people of limited experience and renown and published by them as their first-ever scientific paper, Albert Einstein being the perfect example. Also, sadly, many eminent researchers have published work which is not of the highest quality. The only role examination of authorship plays is in the search process (as we may, e.g. be concerned to include in a review all papers by an acknowledged expert), not the activity of appraisal, in which only the content matters. The same argument applies to the institution in which a study was conducted. As a general rule, as in other aspects of healthcare, in examining published work the importance of authority is far less than the importance of evidence.

Abstract

The abstract is an important issue for authors, as we shall see in Chapter 23, but not for appraisers, with the exception that we will want the abstract, like the title, to be a clear, accurate reflection of the paper's content.

Literature review

Examination of the literature review section varies depending on the paper. If we are evaluating a systematic review, for example, then this is basically all there is to the paper, and so, our evaluation will be comprehensive. We would expect, in such a paper, that the elements laid out in Chapter 4 will be adhered to with regard to searching, selection and data extraction, as well as a high level of critical appraisal broadly following the scheme set out in this chapter. There are a number of guidelines for the detailed, structured evaluation of systematic reviews, including meta-analyses, and these may be found in the websites at the end of this chapter.

However, where we are evaluating the literature review element of a paper reporting the results of a primary research study, our aims are more modest and focused. The literature review should clearly provide a background and rationale for the undertaking of the study which forms the basis of the report. The best reviews do this in a way which leads the reader through briefly recorded general background information, probably from classic studies in the field, through more detailed discussion of studies which relate more closely to the matter being researched in the authors' own study. By this point, we should expect two things in particular. First, the level of critical evaluation of the studies under discussion should be greater, often relating to weaknesses or gaps in the literature. Second, the rationale for the current study should be clearly set in the context of these weaknesses and gaps in the literature. At this point, we should know exactly why the study is being carried out. As an appraiser, you will need to judge the extent to which the authors have given fair evaluations of previous studies and, in consequence, provided an adequate rationale for why they carried out their own study.

Research question

This should be clearly and unambiguously stated. As an appraiser, this is important, because you will need to decide, later in the review, the extent to which the researchers have successfully addressed and answered this question.

Method

In quantitative research, there is a fairly set format for describing method, and this is used in many qualitative studies also, although more leeway is often present in the latter because there is greater variety in the types of approach used, and these sometimes do not easily conform to the established format. Nevertheless, most reports use the following approach to describing method: design/general approach; sample/sampling; setting; measures and materials; procedure; data analysis; ethics.

In each case, two basic rules apply to appraisal. First, and most basic, is there enough detail for you to appraise adequacy of method? The basic rule of thumb here is that the level of detail given would allow a person with good knowledge of the field to replicate the study with minimal need for other information. Many reports, particularly brief reports in professional and popular journals, fail this basic test of quality, and would usually be excluded from systematic reviews on these grounds, because it would be argued that no adequate view of their worth could be arrived at.

Second, if there *is* sufficient detail, how far have the researchers made appropriate methodological choices. In judging this, as we noted above, you, as an appraiser need to balance how far departures from ideal methodology have undermined our confidence in the results of the study against the practical constraints under which the research was carried out. In taking into consideration the second of these, our judgement should be reasonable and fair, but also stringent. We should, for example, recognise the difference between constraints which can and cannot be overcome. Accordingly, we will be more critical of a study which has a small sample of the population from which it is drawn in a very common patient problem, where the researcher reports that time and resource constraints prevented gaining a larger sample, than a study which has an equally small sample but is of an extremely rare problem. Even if the researchers once again plead lack of time and resource, we will probably feel, all in all, that the second study has more merit, because we will recognise that, however much time and money was thrown at it, we would have to wait for a very long time to overcome the problem of small numbers. In other words, it is fair to criticise

Table 22.1 Methodological issues in critical evaluation.

Design –	Is it appropriate to question being asked?
Sample –	Is there a clear rationale for method and size?

Measures –	Are they:
	    validated and/or adequately described?
	    appropriate to the research question?

Procedure –	Is it appropriate to the question:
	    clearly described?
	    accounts for bias?

Data analysis –	Is a clear rationale provided? Does it permit an examination of the research question?

Ethics –	Has ethical approval been gained?
	    Are the issues clearly described?
	    Are issues of special importance fully discussed?

User involvement –	This is an area of broad concern in research, which has both ethical and methodological implications.

the decisions researchers have made, but our criticism should be sympathetic to what is reasonably (or even theoretically) possible.

We have covered a considerable number of these methodological choices in earlier chapters, and many commentators have devised brief checklists for reviewers to help them address methodological issues. Some of these checklists may be found on the websites or in the further reading at the end of this chapter. However, we have also provided a synopsis of the issues in Table 22.1.

Additionally, there are issues specific to or mainly associated with qualitative and quantitative research, and these are presented in Tables 22.2 and 22.3.

Table 22.2 Methodological issues particularly associated with qualitative research.

Design –	Is a theoretical framework described and justified?
Sample –	Where saturation is used to determine eventual sample, are criteria for determining saturation described?
Measures –	Is an interview guide given?
Procedure –	Is there examination of appropriateness of interviewer behaviour? Is there evidence of reflexivity?
Data analysis –	Were independent raters used? Is there an adequate audit trail including details of all stages of decision making in the examination of transcripts and generation of categories and themes? What provision was made for validation of the data?
Ethics –	Have precautions been taken to protect the identity of participants where sample sizes are small and quote material is used?

Table 22.3   Methodological issues particularly associated with quantitative research.

Design –	Has bias been adequately controlled for?
Sample –	Has a power calculation been performed?
	Was a control group used where appropriate?
	Have randomisation procedures (where appropriate) been adequately applied? (Do all prospective participants have a fair and equal chance of inclusion?)
Measures –	Has a main outcome measure associated with the power calculation been identified?
	Is it indicative of important clinical change?
	Does the sample adequately reflect the target population?
Procedure –	In outcome comparisons, are raters and/or patients and/or clinicians unaware of the treatment allocation (blinded)?
	In clinical outcome studies, do the procedures adequately reflect clinical practice?
	In outcome comparison studies, is there adequate specification of the different treatments (including manualisation and staff training where appropriate)?
Data analysis –	Is the statistical approach optimal?
Ethics –	If treatment is withheld, is there an adequate rationale for this?

User involvement in research

We discussed the matter of patient and public involvement in research in Chapters 2 and 5. However, it should be noted that this issue is also important in judging the quality of published research, even though it rarely finds its way into guidelines about how to assess the quality of research. Thus, we recommend that reviewers ask the following questions when reviewing a research paper: how far were patients and carers involved in all stages of the research? If patients and carers were *not* involved, what implications do these have for the research? If this paper is intended for a general audience, how accessible is the writing to non-specialist readers?

Four broad areas of patient and public involvement in research

Identifying and prioritising research topics
Being part of research advisory groups and steering groups
Undertaking research projects and collecting and analysing data
Reporting and communicating research findings

Results

Once again, clarity is the first issue to be examined here. In particular, if the results section is either so brief or so poorly presented as to obscure understanding, this is a serious failing. This should not, however, be confused with the situation where results are genuinely complicated. The researcher cannot be fairly criticised if our own lack of knowledge is to blame for our lack of understanding. As an appraiser, you have to form a judgement as to whether the researcher could reasonably have made the findings clearer.

Two issues, however, are inexcusable. In quantitative research, considerable amounts of material are often presented in tabular form. These tables must be accurate and transparent. For example, in comparisons between treatments, we expect to see clear, accurate reporting of significance levels and the test values associated with them. We also, crucially, expect to see reporting of tests which proved *non-significant*. In other words, the researchers cannot just cherry pick results which support their ideas and ignore results which refute these ideas *or* which fail to provide a clear conclusion either way. The reason for reporting non-significant findings is related to our discussion in Chapter 14 about rejecting hypotheses and in Chapter 20 about the statistical underpinnings of such decisions.

In qualitative research, the same responsibility for being even-handed in reporting results applies as in quantitative research. Thus, researchers should take particular care to report unusual findings which do not easily fit into emerging themes, or which seem to run contradictory to such themes. A further difficulty, in qualitative research relates to the way reports are often organised. Qualitative researchers often report findings in such a way that they are highly integrated with, for example, the findings of others and discussion of both such findings and the results found by the researchers in their current study. We find this method is sometimes confusing, and suggest an alternative which is likely to be clearer (at least for the novice researcher) in our discussion of report writing in Chapter 23. However, where it is used, a considerable problem arises if it becomes difficult or impossible for the reader to distinguish whether a particular piece of information is derived from the findings of the study being reported, previous studies, assertions by the authors of the current study based on opinion, the literature or theory, or assertions made by others and reported by the authors of the study under examination. Where this problem arises, no fair appraisal can be made of this part of the paper, because we do not know whether we are examining findings or something else. This is a profound shortcoming of any paper. The more it occurs, the weaker the paper. However, as in our comments concerning understanding of complex material in quantitative research, appraisers will want to be clear that it is a shortcoming of reporting rather than a superficial reading which has led them to such a criticism.

Discussion

The job of a good discussion is to set the results of a study into context. This context should relate to work that has gone before, both clinical and research, and to potential clinical and research work in the future. In doing so, the discussion should, like the results, be comprehensive and fair. The job of an appraiser is to form a view as to how far the discussion meets these goals. In particular, you will need to consider the extent to which the discussion section of a paper makes such links in ways which are justified on the basis of the findings reported in the results section. First, the researchers should clearly link findings and discussion. Second, the nature of these links should be valid. In other words, the authors, however wide-ranging their comments, should always make these in a way which allows you to see that there is some clear rationale behind them that can be attributed to what they have found in their study, even if there are many links in the chain. There is no limit to how speculative the researchers can be in their recommendations, but you, as an appraiser, are entitled to comment on how well they have justified such speculations.

As just of couple of examples of how poor reporting in the discussion section can obscure meaning, we will look briefly at inappropriate comment on non-significant findings in quantitative research and inappropriate use of language to imply generalisability in qualitative research. In quantitative research you will occasionally see authors commenting on non-significant results which approach significance (values of, say, $p = 0.07$ or even $p = 0.10$). Typically, authors will report that such findings 'just missed showing significance'. There may be some validity in comments of this kind, but there is an implication here that, in some way or other, these findings might, in another place at another time, have *actually been* significant. Of course there is no reason to assume such a thing. However, whilst such a comment may be excusable, it is much worse if the authors then go on to speculate about the likely clinical importance of such non-significant findings *if they had been significant*. Clearly, we could speculate in such a way without having done the study at all. Indeed, this might actually be safer, because there would not be the spurious suggestion of support from a 'nearly' significant finding.

In qualitative research, a somewhat similar issue arises when researchers talk about their sample results as though they were applicable to the populations from whom they were drawn. Typically, this is done through a particular use of language – employing the third person in an impersonal way in the present tense, when a personal sense in the past tense would be more appropriate. For example, if a researcher writes (as many do) something like: 'young drug users feel their identities are threatened by...', we are implicitly invited to believe that *all* young drug users feel this *all the time*. This is a far more powerful assertion than is warranted from any qualitative study, which, as we have seen in previous chapters, concentrates on detailed examination of individual experiences in small samples, rather than general extrapolations of group phenomena to large populations. Imagine how differently we would react to the following: 'The eight drug users in our study felt their identities were threatened by....' or (maybe even better still): 'The eight drug users in our study *reported they* felt their identities were threatened by....'

In these second and third instances we are not invited by the use of general linguistic expressions to assume some general applicability of the findings. Indeed, specification of the people in the noun phrase ('drug users') by pointing out that it was the eight individuals in our study and to a particular point in time by specifying the study and using the past tense ('felt'), invite us to be conservative in the conclusions we draw. The addition, in the third case, of *'reported they'* further specifies this by noting that we do not have privileged access to the feelings and experience of even this sample, but just to their reports of those feelings and experiences (although many commentators would regard such self reports as being good proxies for the feelings and experiences themselves). Both the second and third examples are conservative in the claims they make from findings in a way which the first example is not. Indeed the linguistic form of this first piece of discussion invites us to believe extravagant claims which are not tied to the data.

Part of setting the results in context, and important in making realistic speculations on the basis of results, is the acknowledgment of weaknesses in the study. It is a sign of a strong report where such weaknesses are comprehensively and honestly reported. In such a case, you, as appraiser, form an opinion as to the extent to which such acknowledged difficulties weaken our confidence in the study's findings. Where weaknesses are not acknowledged, but do exist, you are justified in commenting not only on the weaknesses themselves (if you spot them) but also on the fact that they may have been missed by the researchers themselves.

Conclusion

As you will have seen from this chapter, critical evaluation of research reports is not an exact science. A lot will rely on your skill and experience in examining and commenting on research reports, and this requires practice. However, there have been a number of initiatives to standardise critical appraisal, whether through courses or the provision of structured guidelines. It is a moot point the extent to which such guidelines can supplant research experience, methodological knowledge and appraisal experience. However, we have provided a number of key web addresses below, some of which also describe studies of the effectiveness of standardisation in appraisal. In the next chapter, we examine the research report in more detail, this time from the point of view of the author.

Review questions

Why do we need to judge the quality of a research report?
Why is authorship a poor criterion in judging quality?
Why is it important to consider user involvement when judging quality?
What are the key issues in examining the results and discussion sections of a report?

Exercise

Use this chapter to help you critically appraise a paper (of course!)

Further reading

Greenhalgh, T. (2000) *How to Read a Paper*. London: BMJ Books.

Mays, P. and Pope, C. (1995) Qualitative research: rigour and qualitative research. *BMJ*, 311, 109–112.

Murphy, E., Dingwall, R., Greatbatch, D., Parker, S. and Watson, P. (1998) Qualitative research methods in health technology assessment: a review of the literature [Monograph]. *Health Technology Assessment*, 2(16).

Websites

http://www.phru.nhs.uk/Pages/PHD/resources.htm

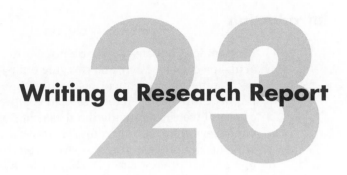

Writing a Research Report

Key points

- The report is a product – help the reader.
- All reports follow a similar general structure.
- The executive summary/lay summary is all most readers will read.
- Do not spend too long on general methodological debate.
- When reporting results:
  - Be clear
  - Be comprehensive
  - Distinguish clearly between results and comment
- A good discussion amplifies the study results, shows the importance of the study results, relates the results to earlier research and theory, admits shortcomings of the study and shows implications for future research and for practice.
- Follow assignment or journal guidelines exactly.
- Write with short words, sentences and paragraphs.
- Use linking sentences to join paragraphs.
- Avoid punctuation you do not understand.
- Write in written English, not spoken English.
- Read work aloud to help with punctuation.

Research for Evidence-Based Practice in Healthcare, Second edition, by Robert Newell and Philip Burnard
© 2011 Robert Newell and Philip Burnard

Introduction

Most undergraduate courses do not require the student to carry out an actual piece of research, and carrying out a small systematic review has become the most frequent research assignment at this level. Reviewing literature has been discussed in Chapters 4 and 22, and a number of useful websites provided in these chapters. All this material is relevant to eventual report writing. However, even at pre-registration level, students are often required to write a research proposal, or an account of a clinical project, and this chapter looks at the presentation of such material.

Many of the points we raised when we look at critical evaluation of published research in Chapter 23 are relevant here. Additionally, we touched on the structure of research reports as early as our examination of how to organise a research project in Chapter 2. However, the current chapter is seen very much from the viewpoint of the research report writer, and so we are concerned here mostly with structure and style, rather than content. In this chapter, we will take a broad look at report writing. Probably your main interest and area of concern will be the composition of a student research assignment or dissertation, and so we will focus mainly on these types of product. Even so, good quality student dissertations can also become disseminated widely, both locally, in your own trust, or even through publication in professional and academic journals. Of course, it may seem that publication is something way beyond your grasp at the moment, but, in our experience, many students (particularly those who already have some clinical experience) produce material which is important to their colleagues, and it is vital that this information is not lost to the clinical community. If you have a product like this, it becomes an ethical responsibility to disseminate it appropriately.

Help the reader

You may have noticed we have now referred twice to the idea of your research report as a product, and we encourage you strongly to think of it in this way, as a completed thing intended for the market place. If your mind is always on the people who will eventually read it, you will communicate much better. If you do *that*, your work will command more influence and respect because more people will read it and find it relevant, because they will see that you have taken care to make it appropriate to them. In considering the reader, you will want to take account of two different things: who is the reader and how can you help them to read your report. When you consider who the reader is, you will write not only in a style which is appropriate, but also with a writing style which you expect will appeal to them. In almost all report writing, this will be a formal writing style. When you try to consider how to help them read the report, you will write in ways which make the report easy to read, understand and remember, and which avoids distracting elements, including errors of grammar, punctuation and so on. This chapter is mainly concerned with structure. However, style is of paramount importance in helping the reader, because familiarity eases the reading process. Teaching writing style could be the subject of many books, and we recommend a couple of the best at the end of this chapter. However, because style is so important, we also give a few basic tips at the close of the chapter which should help your writing style even in the absence of other reading. That said, if you have any doubts about your writing ability, we do strongly advise the further reading.

General structure of the report

All institutions have different preferred layouts for their reports, and these should be followed with slavish devotion. This makes it easier for the examiner to see you have followed the appropriate style, and, in consequence, easier for them to award you marks. The same general rule applies to writing for publication. Even so, there are general structural constraints on reports which we have set out in Figure 23.1.

Prelims

This is editor shorthand for 'preliminaries', and refers to all the material which comes before the main body of the text. In a student report, you need to be sure title, authorship, acknowledgements, tables of contents

- Prelims
- Executive summary/abstract
- Lay summary
- Background/literature review
- Research questions
- Methods
- Included/excluded studies*
- Results
- Discussion
- Recommendations
- References and appendices

*for systematic reviews only

Figure 23.1   General structure of research reports.

and figures are all handled in accordance with your institution guidelines. Over and above that, our comments in Chapters 2 and 22 about clear, relevant titling also apply. Some institutions (and journals) ask for a subtitle and keywords. These are opportunities for you to expand on the information given in your title, specifying further what the report is about.

Executive summary/abstract

Abstract writing is an art. The researcher needs to convey a considerable amount of information, to the reader, in a very few words (normally, not more than about 400 but sometimes considerably fewer). As with the title, every word counts in an abstract. Many research paper search-engines on the internet list only a title and an abstract for any given research project. The fellow-researcher looking at the abstract has to decide whether or not this is a report that he or she needs to obtain and read. The abstract, then, is the 'shop window' for the study.

Abstracts are also included with papers published in refereed journals. Again, the point of them is to guide the reader in answering the question: 'do I want to read this paper'. And again, every word must count and the author is given only a very few words in which to summarise his or her paper. Most readers will be particularly interested in the findings of the study and, as a general rule, a summary of the findings should be the largest part of the abstract.

The writing of an abstract is one of the final tasks for the researcher. It cannot be written until the project is complete because, until then, the findings will not be clear. Because the writing of the abstract takes place late in the project (or, in the case of a journal paper, once the paper has been written) there is sometimes a temptation to write it quickly. The competent researcher, though, knowing the importance of the abstract, will spend time in making sure that it exactly meets the requirement of summarising the work that he or she has done.

The abstract or executive summary is the only part of the report that most people (apart from, say, an examiner) will ever read. To get your message over, you need to have all the important information from the report in this section. Cut every needless word in each sentence, even if it makes the results a bit telegraphic, and ensure all important findings are reported here. Some educational institutions and journals allow abstracts to be written in incomplete sentences, in which case, take full advantage of this to save even more words. It is usually best to follow the structure of the full report precisely in the abstract. Finally, stay within the word limit, especially if writing for publication in a journal. If you go over, they will almost certainly send it back. Similarly, all higher education institutions apply penalties to assignments which exceed the word limit, and some specify word limits for particular sections, such as the abstract, again applying penalties to offenders.

Lay summary

There is some debate over the status of the lay summary in research reports. It is sometimes suggested that no such summary is needed, as all our writing (and, in particular, the executive summary) should be simple and accessible in style. Whilst there is merit to this suggestion, there is, equally, little doubt that specialist readers (including policy makers and clinicians as well as researchers) are more interested in technical detail than most members of the public. There is no reason why this latter group should have to wade through such detail to get at the key messages. Also, executive summaries are often written for what is often called an 'educated readership' – a term which we take to mean people with a good working knowledge of the English language and good general knowledge. Clearly, not all members of the public will meet these criteria, but we should also be aiming to reach these potential users of the research.

Therefore, in our view, lay summaries are important, even though not all funding bodies, publishers, or academics setting and marking student assignments insist on them. A good lay summary should be easily understandable to all, but avoid talking down to the reader. Most importantly, it should not dilute or simplify the findings and implications of a study to such an extent that the resulting messages are simple but misleading.

Key features of a lay summary

Short simple words
Short, single clause sentences
Clear statements of all elements of the research
Technical detail only included if essential to understanding
All main findings included
Discussion contains accurate key messages

Lay summaries (and executive summaries) are also often published in translated form to reflect the main relevant languages other than English. Of course, this is rarely within the resources of a student undertaking a research assignment.

Background/literature review

Remember the structure we described in Chapter 23, where general material receives less coverage in the report than papers which are focal to the research question? In writing a report, this is particularly important, because you will be working within a word limit and will, therefore, have to reach a decision regarding how much space to devote to each study you review. Readers of the review will expect you, at the end of this section, to offer a justification for why you are carrying out your own study, and this is most easily done by pointing to an area of clinical need and to a gap in current research. The literature review is the place to do this. In consequence, save up space to devote to studies which point to the need for your own. Additionally, where studies are weak, this is an opportunity for you to show the examiner your critical appraisal skills and thus gain marks. Accordingly, it is worth picking a couple of weak studies to review in more detail, provided that they are relevant to your own study.

Research questions

Ensure that the reader can clearly see what you intended to investigate. The entire method section should reflect the question, and so this question should be so unambiguous that it is obvious how parts of the method relate to it. Moreover, the question should be capable of being answered, both within the time constraints of the project, and, in principle. Usually, the matter of whether a question can, in principle, be answered relates to the scope of the question. For example, a question which asked 'what is the impact of guidelines on clinical practice?' is probably unanswerable in principle both because its scope is so vast (What guidelines? What practice? What practitioners?), but also because we do not have a clear idea from the question of what is meant by impact and it may be difficult, in practice, to arrive at a definition of impact which all would agree on.

Methods

As discussed in Chapter 22, this material should usually be presented under the conventional headings of design/general approach; sample/sampling; setting; measures; procedure; data analysis; ethics and we refer you to that chapter for detailed discussion. As a report writer, you need to demonstrate to the reader that the choices you have made in terms of method are appropriate to the question being asked and will lead to a useful answer being found. You need, therefore, to provide evidence of your awareness of the issues of method examined in particular in Sections 2 and 3 of this book. However, you have a relatively small space in which to do this, so you will often want to use signposts such as references to methodological books or papers which have used similar methods to answer similar questions, in order to demonstrate your awareness of these issues to the reader in as few words as possible.

This constraint applies particularly when writing for publication. In a student assignment, you are likely to have a more generous word limit, particularly if the assignment is a research proposal, rather than a report of an actual study. Here you have a chance to show the examiner your understanding in more depth, possibly by giving a more extended rationale for the methodological choices you have made. This is similar to the process involved when writing a proposal for funding, where the funding body will want to be assured of the rationale behind the applicant's approach to the research question. If your lecturers have themselves written such proposals, they may be prepared to show them to you, and the way in which they have outlined methodological choices should be a good model for this aspect of the report assignment.

One topic which we suggest you avoid unless it is specifically asked for in the assignment is the prolonged discussion of *general* issues of methodology. In other words, do not go into a long description of the history, theoretical underpinnings and overall applicability of, say, grounded theory or RCTs. This kind of debate is best left for master's dissertations or PhD theses. At pre-registration and undergraduate level, you can usually confine yourself to an examination of why grounded theory or RCT is appropriate to answering *your* research question. As with all other sections of the description of method, this is best achieved by detailed description of what will be done in your study and why.

If your study is a systematic review, exactly the same issues apply, with the proviso that they refer to secondary sources of data (i.e. text materials such as research reports) rather than to primary research. Thus, an exact description of the search and review process should be given. Examples of the structure of systematic review reporting are given on the CRD website at the end of the chapter.

Included/excluded studies

This element of the report applies to systematic reviews only and forms part of the method section of such review studies. It is essential in such reports to give a rationale for why certain studies or categories of study have been excluded from the literature review. Additionally, in large, published reviews, it is common to list all the excluded studies. If your assignment is a report of a systematic review, check whether your institution requires a list of excluded studies. Even if they do not, if it is practical to do so, you may want to consider such a list, as it demonstrates thoroughness of reporting. Lists of excluded papers are definitely *not* required in reporting the literature review of an empirical research study.

Results

Once again – help the reader. We have outlined a number of important issues regarding reporting of results in the previous chapter. As a report

> Be clear – make sure your tables and text are understandable to people other
>   than yourself
> Be comprehensive – do not report just significant findings
> Distinguish clearly between results and comment

Figure 23.2   Issues in results reporting.

author, you will want to take account of these, and we have provided a synopsis in Figure 23.2.

Additionally, remember that readers are helped if you split up the text in a way which helps their attention. This will be particularly useful in the results section, where the material is often complex. In quantitative research, where many of the results are numerical, you have the opportunity to break up the text with tables and graphs. Whilst these can be very helpful, it is important to be aware that their main aim is to aid clarity, and the use of very complex tables, or graphs which include colour and patterns may have the opposite effect. As an author, you should try and strike a balance between text and graphics in such a way as to aid the reader's concentration. Having said that, there is often quite complex numerical information that can *only* be presented in tabular form in a report, because presenting it as text would be repetitive and take up a great deal of space. Finally, everything you report should be there for a reason. For example, the main reason for reporting percentages is to give a sense of the relationship between proportions of responses, particularly when the numbers involved are large or we are being asked to consider relationships between frequencies of response from respondent groups of different sizes. However, it is very common in student essays to see percentages reported for very small respondent groups. It is really not necessary to give results like 3 (30%) in a total respondent group of 10. This kind of reporting adds nothing to our understanding and, arguably, detracts from it by creating a spurious air of scientific accuracy which is not really present in small samples.

In qualitative research, a similar need to guide the reader through the material exists, although the problems involved are slightly different. In quantitative research, we have a situation where the method of presentation (mainly numbers) may be unfamiliar to readers and this may impede understanding. In qualitative research, exactly the reverse situation may apply – the fact that the results are mainly text may draw the reader into reading them in the same way they would read any other kind of text, yet that may be a poor tactic in reading the results of a scientific study, where the meaning of words may be specific and unusual, or may itself be the subject of debate and analysis. It is the job of the author of a report of qualitative research to be particularly careful of the way in which words are used, and to signpost to the reader where words have specific and unusual meanings.

Issues of presentation of results also apply to qualitative research. Because the *amount* of text is generally greater in a qualitative than in a quantitative report, the need to organise the reader's attention is of special importance. It is difficult for readers to mentally organise large amounts of quote material which is reported without comment under a particular theme heading. The reader needs orientating to why such quotes are illustrative of that category, and this is best done by breaking up quote material by commentary which offers a synopsis of related material under a particular theme, tying the quotes together. On the other hand, the use of synopses alone is problematic, because the reader is asked to take on faith the relationship between the respondents' original responses and the emergent themes. As in quantitative research, a balance needs to be struck between quote material and commentary in a way which presents results as faithfully as possible whilst retaining the reader's attention. Finally, as we noted in Chapters 11 and 22, qualitative researchers often include elements of discussion and comment in their results sections. If you do so, be clear the reader can understand from your writing the point at which results end and comment begins. The more you blur results and comment, the more you take the risk that the respondent's voice will not emerge with the clarity you would wish.

Discussion

A good discussion will contain at least the elements outlined in Figure 23.3. Indeed, some journals and many assignment guidelines insist on them.

Amplifying the study results is basically an opportunity for you to say a little more about what the results mean, in lay terms. Typically, this is an element of the discussion we believe can usefully be incorporated into the results section in qualitative research, because it does not lead to the confusion which can arise from including large amounts of theoretical and other comment in the results section. In quantitative research, however, it is very much the tradition that this recounting of

---

Amplification of the study results
Importance of the study results
Relationship of the results to earlier research and theory
Shortcomings of the study
Implications for research
Implications for practice

Figure 23.3 Elements of discussion.

the meaning of the results in *words* rather than figures of tables forms the first part of the discussions section. This, then, leads naturally into a description of what is important about the findings, typically describing how they might change our understanding of the topic under investigation.

Part of this process involves an examination of how the present study's findings fit in with what we understand about the topic already, with reference to the appropriate literature. This is a good opportunity for students to demonstrate their ability to synthesise academic material, and is worth paying a lot of attention to, because this synthetic ability is highly valued by examiners and leads to high marks. Demonstrating the place of your study findings within the broader body of knowledge shows your understanding of the field of study at an advanced level.

Part of the point of science is that it is a community of knowledge, and report writing is a key element of that community. In turn, the willingness to open oneself to the scrutiny of peers is part of that community endeavour, and includes the open admission of error. Accordingly, as an author, you should examine your study closely for methodological problems and report these fully. In the context of a student assignment, the ability to recognise these difficulties in taken as a sign of the strength of the student's work. Naturally, if you can defend sub-optimal methodological choices, suggest reasons why these were inevitable or did not compromise the research results, and offer credible alternative approaches for the future, so much the better.

Finally, our research should have consequences. Hopefully, you have already explained the general consequences of your research for the field of study, but it is also good practice to note how the results might lead to further research and to changes in practice. You may feel that a student assignment is unlikely to have such far-reaching implications, but it is surprising how many changes to practice have begun with small pilot studies. Just remember to be realistic and provide evidence from your study to back up your assertions.

Recommendations

Some assignment guidelines ask that implications for practice and research are presented as a separate recommendations section. If this is the case, take care not to repeat material from the discussion section. It can be useful to set out a recommendations section in a structured form, with each recommendation followed by the relevant evidence. See Figure 23.4 for an example.

References and appendices

These should follow the guidelines for any piece of academic work. However, in research reporting, you may also use the appendices to

> Recommendation 9: New patients attending for surgery should be introduced to a theatre practitioner who will have overall responsibility for their care during their stay in theatre.
>
> Rationale: Our study found patients who were introduced to a theatre practitioner who they know would take charge of their care reported less anxiety during the perioperative period.
>
> *Note*: this example is for illustrative purposes, and not the results of an actual study.

Figure 23.4   Example of structured recommendation reporting.

include material which would be helpful to other researchers, even though it is not essential to an understanding of the report (e.g. interview schedules, specially designed questionnaires, patient information sheets).

Basic style tips

Follow house style guides: This is a 'must' whether you are writing a student project or a paper for journal publication. It is so easy to refer to the assignment guidelines, and yet many students do not. Sometimes, as much as 20% of marks is awarded for appropriate presentation and referencing. These marks are the easiest to get, because they require no actual thought at all. You just follow the rules! In the case of journals, they all have *ITAs* – Instructions to Authors – which outline the journal's presentation requirements – most of which are available on the web. The *British Medical Journal's* ITA is one of the most comprehensive, and its web address is given at the end of the chapter. Please do not dismiss it because it is medical. It is a great guide to clear, concise academic writing. An added bonus is that the general word limit for *BMJ* papers is 2000 words – about the size of many student assignments.

Write with short words, sentences and paragraphs. Good writing is clear, and clear writing is expressed in short units of thought, making it easier for readers to keep each idea in memory as they read. We have commonly heard from students who, having written long, rambling sentences, say their lecturers have asked them to write *longer* sentences. This is poor advice, and we suspect that what those lecturers really wanted was more development of an idea or argument. Write sentences which are no longer than needed to express an idea. If an idea gets complex, write more sentences, not longer ones.

Use linking sentences to join each paragraph to the next. This helps the reader to keep reading, because they experience a general forward motion of the text and its arguments, rather than a series of jumps.

Avoid the colon and semicolon, except in lists. Few people understand the use of the colon and semicolon and most times the full stop will do just as well or better. Use of the colon and semicolon also leads to long, complex sentences. There is no use of the colon or semicolon in this chapter, except in lists, and probably only about a dozen or so uses in this whole book, which runs at about 90 000 words. Do you miss them?

Report writing is a formal exercise, and formal written English differs from informal written English (tabloid newspapers, magazines) and spoken English. Sometimes, the formality makes formal written English more difficult to read, but this is usually because this type of English is more dense – the writer is often trying to pack in a lot of information in a comparatively short space. What you are reading in this book is an example of formal written English, but at the low end of formal. Columns in *Nursing Times* are at the top end of informal written English, clinical papers in *Nursing Times* are at the low end of formal English, research papers about in the middle. Research papers in *Journal of Advanced Nursing* are at the top end of formal English. Student papers are best pitched at the middle range of formal written English, although anywhere in the formal range is acceptable.

With this in mind, write in complete thoughts and complete sentences. All sentences should contain an active verb (look at a style book or grammar book if you do not understand what we are on about). We also generally recommend writing in the third person. In qualitative research, there is now a trend towards writing in the first person, partly as a recognition of the role of the researcher in shaping the process of the research encounter. However, we find that student writing in the first person has two unfortunate consequences. First, the general tone of the writing becomes too informal and colloquial for report writing, and, second, the writer often does not stay in the first person, but swaps back and forward between first and third, sometimes, in surprising places. First person report writing is an advanced skill.

Do not connect two sentences with a comma. Again, you may need to look at a grammar book to get the point here. However, in our experiences, the best guide to modern English sentencing and punctuation is to read aloud what you have written. If you do this sensitively, you will *know* that it should be a full stop, not a comma and so on.

Review questions

What is the general structure of the research report?
Is a lay summary always needed? When it is, what are its main features?
What are the key issues in reporting results?

Exercise

Identifying the implications for research and practice is an element of research writing students often find difficult.

If you are currently undertaking a research project, consider all the likely findings and ask what would be the next questions you would ask as a result of these findings and what would change in what you would do as a practitioner.

If you are not yet doing a research project yourself, read a piece of published research in which the writer has *not* identified implications for research and practice. Once again, ask what would be the next questions you would ask as a result of their findings and what would change in what you would do as a nurse.

Further reading

Burnard, P. (1995) *Writing for Health Professionals: A Manual for Writers*. Cheltenham: Nelson Thornes.

Holton, D. and Fisher, E. (1999) *Enjoy Writing Your Science Thesis or Dissertation*. London: Imperial College Press.

Newell, R. (2001) Writing academic papers: a guide for prospective authors. *Intensive and Critical Care Nursing*, 17, 110–116.

Thomas, S.A. (2000) *How to Write Health Sciences Papers, Dissertations and Theses*. Edinburgh: Churchill Livingstone.

Walcott, H. (2001) *Writing up Qualitative Research*. London: Sage.

Getting Research into Practice

Introduction

We have emphasised throughout this book the idea that healthcare research should be, at root, about effective patient care. One important consequence of this idea is that the results of research should be made

Research for Evidence-Based Practice in Healthcare, Second edition, by Robert Newell and Philip Burnard
© 2011 Robert Newell and Philip Burnard

available to practitioners, to patients and the public. It may seem an unlikely proposition that you, the lone researcher, can exert any influence on practice, and indeed most research these days is done in groups, but all research starts somewhere, and this includes the work of undergraduate students and lone researchers in clinical practice, as well as patients and carers seeking answers to healthcare issues which affect their lives. Moreover, work you will have done in literature searching and evaluation is itself of immense potential importance to others. Traditionally, healthcare researchers, like other academics, have published their work in academic and professional journals. However, this method of dissemination is known to be one of the least effective at reaching other people in clinical practice and likewise one of the least useful approaches to effecting change. Because healthcare practitioners have so much power to influence the way in which care is practiced, the rest of this chapter talks about how you can reach and influence clinical and managerial colleagues effectively.

The nature of the change process

Introducing change in clinical practice is helped if we have a knowledge of the process of change as it relates to innovative ideas. E.M. Rogers (1983) introduced the notion of *diffusion of innovation* to describe how an innovation is taken up by members of society over time. Rogers suggested that people would be grouped in terms of how quickly they would incorporate some new device, activity of idea into their way of life. At one end of the continuum, *innovators* are adventurous people who are open to change and have the resources to take up new devices or ideas almost as soon as they are available. They account for about 5% of the population. *Early adopters* see advantages to taking up the innovation at an early stage and account for a further 10%. The next two groups (*early majority* and *late majority* [35% each]) represent categories into which most of us fall, and take up innovations as they gain wider acceptance, with the early majority being more open to change, and the later majority more sceptical as to the value of change and seeking to eliminate risk from the change process). Finally, *laggards* (15%) resist change for as long as possible.

Although Rogers put forward no specific evidence in support of this categorisation, surveys have suggested that this range of proposed responses actually conforms very well to the pattern of diffusion of many new ideas in society. It is worth considering people we know, not just from clinical practice, in Rogers's terms. We have no doubt you will be able to place your friends and colleagues easily within one or other of the categories in the previous paragraph, both with regard to their views of specific innovations and of innovation generally. The influence of personal characteristics is one element which affects the diffusion of change. The other major factor is how accessible the change is to those for whom its use is intended. Accessibility can be governed by a number of factors. For example, in the first edition of this book, we noted that television was an almost entirely accepted technology in our society, and so barriers in terms of individual readiness to change were unlikely to be critical to the introduction of a new form of television. Despite this, the 'flat screen' television was still (about 5 years ago) the preserve of only a minority of consumers (presumably those in the innovator and early adopter categories), and we suggested that the main barrier to diffusion was likely to have been cost (with consequent limiting of accessibility) rather than reservations over the technology. As we write today, the cost of flat screen televisions has plummeted, removing this potential barrier, and such TVs are now the norm, with cathode ray televisions now extinct and probably as distant a memory to as many of our readers as the valve wireless is to people of our generation.

The analogy with healthcare, however, remains clear. If an innovation is compromised in terms of accessibility, either because of cost or other limiting factors (lack of appropriately trained staff; time-consuming nature of the intervention), then this places a considerable constraint on its diffusion within healthcare. Moreover, in healthcare, because innovation is common, the resource constraints on its adoption are influenced by the effect of competition on resources, as many different changes (some of dubious pedigree in terms of evidence) are introduced in quick succession, all requiring implementation by busy clinicians.

Effectiveness of interventions to get research into practice

We said at the beginning of this chapter that journal publications are likely to be an *ineffective* way of introducing change into clinical practice. The reason for this is simple – few clinicians read much at all to do with their work, and fewer still read the academic journals in which researchers likely to publish. This is a problem of preaching to the choir – innovators essentially diffusing only to other innovators. We know that journal publication is comparatively ineffective because there have been numerous studies into the effectiveness of a range of different ways of effecting healthcare change.

The Centre for Reviews and Dissemination (CRD) has published an *Effective Healthcare* bulletin on this topic (NHS Centre for Reviews and Dissemination, 1999) which details the tactics which are likely and unlikely to prove useful. Whilst the bulletin is over 10 years old now, and makes comparatively little reference to non-medical research and practice, the general points made are unlikely to have changed, and the CRD review is still the best synopsis of the issues surrounding getting research into practice. It concluded that, despite the incomplete nature of investigation of attempts to get research into practice, it was still possible to reach some conclusions about what strategies were likely to be effective.

First, a clear dissemination and implementation strategy should be devised on the basis of a diagnostic analysis within the organisation. Evidence suggested that the following components should be incorporated into this analysis.

Components of a diagnostic analysis for change implementation

- Identification of all groups likely to be affected
- Assessment of characteristics of the change that might influence its implementation
- Assessment of the target group (readiness to change? Other individual/group factors)
- Identification of external barriers to change
- Identification of enabling factors

This analysis would then inform broad-based approaches to implementation. Such broad-based approaches have been found to be more effective than single interventions. The types of intervention included in the approach should once again be targeted to the group to be affected and to the nature of the change.

Components of getting research into practice where there is some evidence of effectiveness include educational outreach; clinical reminders; use of local opinion leaders; audit with feedback. The final two approaches were less consistent in terms of the evidence for their effectiveness. Whilst the degree and consistency of the evidence for these interventions is variable, three factors emerge. First, none is useful in all situations. Second, there seems to be a clear distinction between all these approaches and the less effective results available from dissemination alone. Third, all these studies involve *active* measures of one kind or another to engage with the target group. Thus, educational outreach generally involves visits to the clinical areas by promoters of the change. Reminders need to be available to the clinician close to or at the point of contact with patients. Local opinion leaders exert positive influence by virtue of their endorsement of an initiative. Audit and feedback are continuing activities which demonstrate to clinicians their performance relative to the desired change.

Interestingly, dissemination of educational materials alone has been found to be ineffective in promoting change in clinical practice. This includes studies of clinical practice guidelines. Similarly, the evidence around continuing quality initiatives (which have enjoyed great popularity in the NHS), is very mixed. In the CRD review, whilst uncontrolled studies showed effectiveness for such initiatives, no controlled studies showed such effects. Clinicians seeking to disseminate by such means should consider their local circumstances very carefully in order to see whether there is any element of these circumstances which would justify such tactics, given the absence of strong evidence of effectiveness.

Looking at more global factors in influencing change, the Getting Research into Policy and Practice (GRIPP) initiative has promoted an overall approach to dissemination and implementation strategies. This approach is based on the diffusion model and begins with development of the research question, including such ideas as involving clinicians and policy makers in shaping research questions, in order to increase their likely relevance to care. Further stages in the GRIPP process closely follow the stages in the diffusion model presented above. Some specific examples and case studies, mainly from the field of public health are available at the websites at the end of this chapter. For a number of reviews of effective organisation of care (including a variety of approaches to getting research and evidence into practice), see the following site on the Cochrane Collaboration library: http://www.cochrane.org/reviews/en/topics/61_reviews.html

Barriers to implementation

Of the stages in the diffusion model, the identification of barriers merits special attention. In the first place, this topic has been considerably studied in healthcare. Secondly, it is the issue of barriers which most researchers and clinicians seeking to implement changes in practice will find occupy most of their time. We both remember, even as student nurses, frustration at ingrained, ritualistic practices which we would have liked to change, and remember equally well the wide range of reasons put forward by colleagues as to why no change was possible. We are sure people reading this book will have felt the same on many occasions.

As early as 1987, Funk *et al.* (1991) developed and validated a scale which identified factors likely to impede the adoption of research in nursing. This scale has since been used in other health professions as well. This scale (the BARRIERS scale) consists of four components, which are linked, once again to aspects of the diffusion model:

- Characteristics of the adopter (nurses' values, skills, awareness)
- Characteristics of the organisation (perceived barriers and limitations of the setting
- Characteristics of the innovation: the qualities of the research
- Characteristics of the communication: presentation and accessibility of the research

Each component contains a number of specific statements which, taken together, allow a detailed picture of barriers and facilitators of research within an organisation to be gained. For example, under the category of *characteristics of the adopter*, such issues as whether the HCP sees the value of research for practice and for herself, whether she believes changing practice will be beneficial, whether there is a documented need for change, are explored in the context of the organisation, giving a picture of the organisational perception of barriers to change. The existence of a validated scale is potentially useful in allowing those who seek to introduce change to gain an accurate perception of perceptions of barriers to research within their organisation. This is an important contribution to the diagnostic analysis and, therefore, to the effective introduction of change.

Creating clinical guidelines: a change strategy in your organisation?

Given that dissemination of clinical guidelines alone seems to be of limited use, one might question the value of devising them in the first place. Certainly, medical and healthcare practice are currently informed by a plethora of such guidelines. Moreover, there is little doubt that they have great potential to standardise and enhance the quality of care. Once again, the issue is one of utilising an appropriate strategy for implementation, rather than simply making the guideline available. An earlier review (Effective Healthcare, 1994) stressed the importance of local circumstances, active educational interventions and patient-specific reminders rather than a blanket approach to dissemination. In such circumstances, the potential of guidelines grows considerably, and many of the lessons of both Effective Healthcare bulletins have been incorporated into NHS initiatives aimed at improving care through guidelines. Currently, major guidelines in the NHS are co-ordinated by the National Institute for clinical excellence (NICE) and its collaborating centres. The collaborating centre for nursing guidelines is based at the RCN Institute in Oxford. To date, major nursing guidelines exist in the management of just a few nursing interventions, including management of wound infection and leg ulceration.

However, many hospitals and units have used the introduction of local guidelines to systematise nursing care, particularly when clinical uncertainty as to best practice exists. We recommend you examine http://www.ferne.org/Lectures/GLDiffintro0402.htm for an excellent web lecture on use of guidelines. The major steps in the process of creating guidelines are summarised in Figure 24.1 and key issues discussed below.

As you can see, guideline development relies on evidence, and this has been covered in some detail in Chapters 4 and 22, which deal with

Scoping
Devising a workplan
Forming a guideline development group
Developing the clinical question(s)
Identifying and appraising the literature
Arriving at decisions
Making recommendations
Agreeing audit procedures
Writing the guidelines
Consulting stakeholders
Updating guidelines

Figure 24.1   Steps in guideline creation.

literature searching and appraisal, respectively. The notion of scoping is also similar to one of the activities required in literature searching, and with the broadly similar aim of identifying the nature and extent of the problem and its associated evidence base. As guideline creation typically involves a wide group of stakeholders, the second stage involves identifying group members, negotiating roles, specifying the tasks to be performed and agenda setting.

Clinical questions are derived from the scoping exercise and are similar in form to the questions that guide systematic reviews (see Chapter 4). The development of recommendations is derived from appraisal of the literature, but will include issues of prioritisation, implementation and audit of compliance and effectiveness. Once again, because of the broad nature of the guideline creation process and the many groups involved with the process, writing the eventual guideline is typically an iterative process, with the writers seeking feedback from all stakeholders and reviewing the way the guideline is written in the light of that feedback, in order to increase the usability and acceptability of the guideline to those for whom it is intended. These issues relate to content as well as style, because stakeholders may well have suggestions about which aspects of a guideline are more and less applicable to the local context. Finally, the team should set an agenda for updating, in the expectation that new research will become available and that the local context within which the guidelines operate will change.

And finally. . .

This is pretty much the end of this book, and we hope you have found it useful. We have tried to stress four things throughout. First, that research and the evidence-based care that springs from it are practical undertakings. As a result of this, whilst we hope that reading this book alone will help you in your understanding and conduct of research, we also want very much for you to go out and get involved, in whatever way best fits with and informs your clinical practice. This brings us to our second point, the one this particular chapter has been all about – that research is *about* clinical practice. It is, in our view, vitally important to gather evidence which will guide our activities with patients. Third, research is complex and difficult, but no more so than many clinical tasks. And finally, that, even though it is complex and difficult, it is entirely possible for you, as a clinician, to become involved and to truly make a difference to the care of your patients. Remember the story about eating an elephant, and just take it a bit at a time.

> ### Review questions
>
> What are the key elements of the diffusion model?
> What are the components of a diagnostic analysis?
> What are the major barriers to change?

Exercise

Identify some area of practice which you know would benefit from changing in line with best evidence. Examine the stages of the diffusion model and conduct your own diagnostic analysis of the implementation of change in this area of practice.

References

Funk, S.G., Champagne, M.T., Wiese, R.A. and Tornquist, E.M. (1991) BARRIERS: the barriers to research utilization scale. *Applied Nursing Research*, 4(1), 39–45.

NHS Centre for Reviews and Dissemination (1999) Getting evidence into practice. *Effective Health Care*, 5(1), 1–16.

Rogers, E.M. (1983) *Diffusion of Innovations*. New York: Free Press.

Further reading

Clark, J.E. and Clifford, C. (2004) *Getting Research into Practice: A Health Care Approach*. Edinburgh: Churchill Livingstone.

Francke, A.L., Smit, M.C., de Veer, A.J.E. and Mistiaen, P. (2008) Factors influencing the implementation of clinical guidelines for health care professionals:

a systematic meta-review. *BMC Medical Informatics and Decision Making*, 8(38). Available online at http://www.biomedcentral.com/1472-6947/8/38.

Haines, A. and Donald, A. (2002) *Getting Research Findings into Practice*. London: BMJ Books.

Kelly, M.P., Speller, V. and Meyrick, J. (2004) *Getting Evidence into Practice in Public Health*. London: Health Development Agency.

Websites

http://www.ferne.org/Lectures/GLDiffintro0402.htm

http://www.gserve.nice.org.uk/niceMedia/pdf/evidence_into_practice.pdf

http://www.popcouncil.org/pdfs/frontiers/FR_FinalReports/Interregional_GRIPPSuppl.pdf

http://www.shef.ac.uk/scharr/ir/units/resprac/index.htm

http://www.socstats.soton.ac.uk/choices/workshop/

http://www.who.int/bulletin/volumes/85/6/07-042531/en/index.html

Appendix 1
Research Log

An editable version of this log will be available from this book's web page

Title
Initial thoughts (now)

Reflection (after reading relevant material)

Aims and objectives
Initial response (now)

Reflection (after reading relevant material)

Literature review
Initial response (now)

Reflection (after reading relevant material – Chapters 4 and 22)

Research question
Initial response (now)

Reflection (after reading relevant material)

Sample and sampling approach
Initial response (now)

Reflection (after reading relevant material – Chapter 6 and 13)

Materials and measures
Initial response (now)

Reflection (after reading relevant material)

Data collection
Initial response (now)

Reflection (after reading relevant material – chapters which discuss specific research methods)

Procedures
Initial response (now)

Reflection (after reading relevant material – chapters which discuss specific research methods, but especially Chapters 15, 16 and 17)

Data analysis
Initial response (now)

Reflection (after reading relevant material – Chapters 11 and 20)

Ethical issues
Initial response (now)

Reflection (after reading relevant material – Chapter 5)

Resources needed
Initial response (now)

Reflection (after reading relevant material)

Dissemination
Initial response (now)

Reflection (after reading relevant material – Chapters 23 and 24)

Timetable

Appendix 2
List of Useful Websites
(In Order of Citation)

http://www.bun.kyoto-u.ac.jp/~suchii/holmes_1.html
Website using Sherlock Holmes as an example of inductive and deductive reasoning (Honestly).

http://www.fortunecity.com/greenfield/grizzly/432/rra2.htm
Nice website giving synopses of qualitative and quantitative approaches to research, including different methodological approaches.

http://www.cochrane.org
Homepage of the Cochrane Collaboration – contains a wide range of information and guidance.

http://www.york.ac.uk/inst/crd/
Centre for Reviews and Dissemination website – contains links to their publications and advice on systematic reviewing.

http://www2.carleton.ca/secretariat/policies/the-ethical-conduct-of-research/
US University web page outlining policies for research ethics. Useful introduction to the detailed consideration of issues which arise from the basic ethical principles of autonomy, beneficence and justice.

http://www.nres.npsa.nhs.uk/
The website of the National Research Ethics Service. Contains lots of information about research ethics and the work of ethics committees in the UK.

http://www.dh.gov.uk/en/Researchanddevelopment/A-Z/
Researchgovernance/index.htm
NHS research governance website.

http://www.mrc.ac.uk/Newspublications/Publications/
Ethicsandguidance/index.htm
Medical Research Council website's research ethics pages. Extensive re-
source, with much information relevant to nurses.

http://www.depauloresearch.com/sampsize.htm
Interesting web article on sample size in qualitative research.

http://hsc.uwe.ac.uk/dataanalysis/qualWhat.asp
Excellent University of West of England site which gives an introduction to qualitative data analysis, including useful exercises. The site is
part of a larger site which also contains lots of other very good intro-
ductory material, including webpages on research topics, including one
on quantitative data analysis (see Chapter 20).

http://chiron.valdosta.edu/whuitt/col/intro/valdgn.html
Great online essay on the topics of external and internal validity, seen
mainly from a psychology standpoint, but entirely relevant to health
care.

http://www.socialresearchmethods.net/kb/sampling.php
Thorough introduction to sampling, with pages on general reliability
and validity. This site also has lots of good material on general research
design issues.

http://www.shef.ac.uk/content/1/c6/06/59/35/Scope%20tutorial%
204.pdf
Free-access online tutorial from a respected UK site, covering hypothesis testing and estimation.

http://www.dssresearch.com/toolkit/spcalc/power_a2.asp
Simple-to-follow power calculation for a number of common experimental approaches.

http://www.csulb.edu/~msaintg/ppa696/696quasi.htm
This site gives a good run down on a variety of quasi-experimental
approaches, often in considerable detail. Although some of the material requires close attention (partly because the examples are not from
health care, and partly because of the language used), this is well worth
the effort.

http://www.phru.nhs.uk/Doc_Links/rct%20appraisal%20tool.pdf
Critical appraisal site with a good, clear checklist for appraisal criteria
for RCTs.

http://clem.mscd.edu/~davisj/prm2/correl1.html#1
Brief descriptions of main concepts of correlational research.

http://psych.umb.edu/faculty/kogan/files/Handouts_
CorrelationalDesigns.pdf
Powerpoint presentation from a US psychology course. This is a very
clear and engaging description of correlation.

www.uiowa.edu/~resmeth/study_questions/sq-descrip-ccomp.html
Website with some exam questions about causal comparative designs
which might give you some food for thought.

http://hsc.uwe.ac.uk/dataanalysis/quantWhat.asp
University of West of England webpages covering quantitative analysis
and statistical appreciation. Very good.

http://www.medicine.ox.ac.uk/bandolier/
Excellent evidence-based health care site. As well as regular reviews,
this site also contains many well-written, accessible authoritative articles on methodological issues relevant to evidence-based practice – just
scroll down the site page to see these.

http://www.bmj.com/cgi/content/full/312/7023/71?view=long&
pmid=8555924
Web publication of British Medical Journal paper introducing the concepts of evidence-based practice and examining common misrepresen-
tations of the EBP initiative. Irritatingly, you can only get straight to
this paper through this link if you are a registered BMJ user. If not, you
need to go through: http://www.ncbi.nlm.nih.gov/pubmed/8555924
then click on the **Full text-FREE/BMJ** button on the right-hand side of
the page.

http://www.cebm.utoronto.ca/practise/formulate/pg2.htm
Canadian EBP website, again with lots of useful downloads.

http://www.cebm.utoronto.ca/practise/formulate/pg2.htm
Canadian EBP website, again with lots of useful downloads.

http://www.phru.nhs.uk/Pages/PHD/resources.htm
Good source of structured guidelines about how to critically appraise a
research paper.

http://www.ferne.org/Lectures/GLDiffintro0402.htm
Great US website. Do not be put off by the fact that the author is a medical practitioner. This site contains a Powerpoint presentation plus a free online lecture (needs Realplayer™ software). We nearly did not write this chapter after seeing this site!

http://www.shef.ac.uk/scharr/ir/units/resprac/index.htm
Clear introduction to the process of getting research into practice from the SCHARR website.

http://www.socstats.soton.ac.uk/choices/workshop/
University of Southampton website which describes the 2001 workshop which gave rise to the Getting Research into Policy and Practice. Contains many useful presentations.

http://www.who.int/bulletin/volumes/85/6/07-042531/en/index.html
World Health Organization online bulletin feature article from 2007 on getting research into practice.

Index

Note: Page numbers with f and t refer to figures and tables.